RANSOM KHANYE

The Green Pharmacy

A Guide to 30 Natural Antibiotics

Cover design by Ransom Khanye

ISBN: 9798872149118

Also available on Amazon, about natural remedies, and by the same author:

1. The Magic Oil: Unleashing the Power of Nature's Remedy - Castor Oil
2. The Magic Oil 2: More Castor Oil Miracles
3. Amazing Natural Remedies: Nature's Medicine Cabinet
4. 101 Castor Oil Recipes for Health and Beauty

FOREWORD

Welcome to "The Green Pharmacy: A Guide to 30 Natural Antibiotics"! In this botanical odyssey, we embark on a journey through the lush landscapes of nature's medicine cabinet, exploring the vibrant world of herbal antibiotics. As you turn the pages of this guide, prepare to discover the untapped potential of green remedies that have been thriving under our noses, awaiting their moment in the spotlight.

In a world where the quest for well-being often leads us to the aisles of pharmacies, "The Green Pharmacy" invites you to step into a realm where healing is as natural as the world around us. Here, each chapter unfolds a new leaf, revealing the incredible powers of 50 natural antibiotics that have been revered by ancient cultures and embraced by modern science.

From the fiery depths of Cayenne Pepper to the soothing embrace of Chamomile, each herb and spice holds a unique tale of healing. Picture a pharmacy where the shelves are lined with vibrant leaves, fragrant blooms, and robust roots—nature's own prescriptions for vitality. Through engaging narratives, practical tips, and real-life examples, this guide aims to empower you to make informed choices about your health, tapping into the green wisdom that has sustained humanity for centuries.

The green in "The Green Pharmacy" symbolizes not just the color of the plants but also the embodiment of life, growth, and renewal. It represents a return to the roots of healing, embracing the wisdom passed down through generations and marrying it with contemporary scientific understanding. This guide is a celebration of the green, the vibrant, and the living—a testament to the profound healing potential that nature graciously offers.

As you navigate the chapters of this guide, you'll encounter not just information but a symphony of words that aims to captivate, educate, and inspire. From the fiery kick of cayenne to the soothing touch of chamomile, each chapter is crafted to be a standalone exploration, inviting you to savor the richness of herbal antibiotics in bite-sized doses.

So, dear reader, fasten your seatbelt for a botanical adventure that promises to transform the way you perceive healing. "The Green Pharmacy" is not just a book; it's your passport to a world where nature's pharmacy beckons, and vibrant well-being is within arm's reach.

Happy reading and welcome to the green revolution!

Sincerely,

Ransom Khanye
Author, "The Green Pharmacy: A Guide to 30 Natural Antibiotics"

Contents

Introduction to Nature's Healing Pharmacy

In the midst of modern medicine's complexity, there is a vibrant and timeless pharmacy waiting to be explored – the world of natural antibiotics. Welcome to "The Green Pharmacy," where the age-old wisdom of healing herbs converges with the latest scientific discoveries to bring you a guide to 30 natural antibiotics.

Picture yourself walking through a lush botanical garden, surrounded by an array of vibrant colors and intoxicating scents. Each plant, a guardian of health, holding within its leaves, roots, or blossoms the potential to heal and protect. This journey isn't just about remedies; it's an exploration of the profound connection between nature and well-being.

In this guide, we transcend the ordinary boundaries of health literature. "The Green Pharmacy" is not just a book; it's an invitation to a holistic experience. As you turn the pages, you'll delve into the depths of ancient traditions, the nuances of herbal alchemy, and the cutting-edge science behind natural antibiotics.

The selection of these 30 natural antibiotics is no arbitrary list; it's a curated collection of botanical wonders chosen for their proven efficacy and diverse applications. Whether you seek immune support, relief from common ailments, or a preventive approach to wellness, this guide has something for everyone

Consider this book your passport to a realm where healing is synonymous with nature's bounty. Each chapter is a doorway into the world of a specific natural antibiotic, revealing its unique properties, historical significance, and practical applications. The goal?

Empowering you to take charge of your well-being with knowledge that transcends conventional medicine.

"The Green Pharmacy" is not just about treating illnesses; it's a celebration of preventive healthcare. By understanding and incorporating these natural antibiotics into your lifestyle, you're not merely addressing symptoms – you're fortifying your body's natural defenses.

Are you ready to embark on a transformative journey? As you step into "The Green Pharmacy," let the exploration begin. Discover the wonders of herbal antibiotics, unlock the secrets of ancient remedies, and embrace a path towards a healthier, more vibrant you.

This isn't just a book; it's a promise – a promise that the pages you're about to turn hold the key to a greener, healthier, and more harmonious life. Welcome to "The Green Pharmacy," where nature's pharmacy becomes your guide to lasting well-being.

1: The Fiery Guardian - Cayenne Pepper (Capsicum annuum) as an Antibacterial

In the vibrant world of herbal antibiotics, one spice stands out as a fiery guardian of health – Cayenne Pepper. The tale of this potent red pepper goes beyond the realms of flavor; it unfolds as a compelling narrative of antibacterial prowess, spanning centuries and cultures.

The Spice that Ignites Health:
Picture this: a bustling market in ancient civilizations, where traders barter not only goods but also the secrets of healing. Among these treasures, the fiery Cayenne Pepper emerges, coveted for its multifaceted benefits. Fast forward to today, and this spice remains a staple in kitchens worldwide, valued not only for its culinary zest but also for its remarkable antibacterial properties.

The Heat That Heals:
Cayenne owes its fiery heat to capsaicin, a potent compound that not only ignites taste buds but also sets ablaze harmful bacteria. As you consume Cayenne Pepper, it activates a cascade of reactions in your body, leading to increased blood circulation, heightened metabolism, and a boost in immune response. This fiery spice becomes a formidable force against bacterial invaders.

Antibacterial Symphony:
Imagine Cayenne Pepper as the conductor of an antibacterial symphony within your body. It orchestrates a series of actions that dismantle bacterial threats. Capsaicin, the spice's active component, has been

scientifically recognized for its ability to inhibit the growth of various bacteria, including strains that can lead to infections.

Practical Tips for Incorporating Cayenne:

1. Morning Elixir:
Start your day with a cleansing elixir. Mix a pinch of Cayenne Pepper with warm water, lemon juice, and a touch of honey. This concoction not only jumpstarts your metabolism but also sets a powerful antibacterial tone for the day.

2. Culinary Zest:
Introduce Cayenne into your daily cooking. Sprinkle it on soups, stews, or roasted vegetables. Not only does it add a fiery kick to your meals, but it also fortifies them with antibacterial properties.

3. Homemade Antibacterial Salve:
Craft a simple antibacterial salve using Cayenne Pepper. Mix a small amount of powdered Cayenne with coconut oil and beeswax. Apply this salve topically to minor cuts or abrasions for a natural antibacterial boost.

4. Spice-infused Teas:
Explore the world of spice-infused teas. Combine Cayenne with ginger, turmeric, and a hint of honey for a soothing, immune-boosting beverage. This not only warms your soul but also provides a bacterial defense mechanism.

Anecdote: The Healing Heat of Grandma's Remedy

In the heart of a small village, nestled between rolling hills, lived Grandma Maria. Her remedy for various ailments was a testament to the healing power of Cayenne Pepper. One winter, when the village was gripped by a seasonal flu, Grandma Maria prepared a fiery brew using Cayenne, honey, and ginger. The villagers, skeptical yet desperate for relief, embraced her remedy. To their astonishment, the potent blend not only provided warmth but also helped ward off the flu.

The story of Grandma Maria's Cayenne concoction spread like wildfire, becoming a cherished tradition in the village. Generations later, the villagers still swear by the healing heat of Cayenne, a testament to the enduring efficacy of this humble spice.

Closing Thoughts:
As we unravel the story of Cayenne Pepper, remember that nature's bounty often holds the solutions we seek. In the case of Cayenne, its fiery essence not only tantalizes our taste buds but also shields us from unseen bacterial threats. Embrace the heat, savor the spice, and let Cayenne Pepper be your fiery ally in the journey toward optimal health.

Sources:
1. O'Neil, C. R., Hanlon, J. T., & Marcum, Z. A. (2010). Adverse effects of herbal and dietary supplements on clinical laboratory test results. Archives of Internal Medicine, 170(16), 1501–1508.
2. Govindarajan, V. S., & Sathyanarayana, M. N. (1991). Capsicum—Production, technology, chemistry, and

quality. Part V. Impact on physiology, pharmacology, nutrition, and metabolism; structure, pungency, pain, and desensitization sequences. Critical Reviews in Food Science & Nutrition, 29(6), 435–474.

3. Bernstein, J. A., Davis, B. P., & Picard, J. K. (2007). Pilot study of the effect of Capsicum frutescens on nasal symptom severity and quality of life in subjects with perennial allergic rhinitis. Journal of Alternative and Complementary Medicine, 13(4), 391–400.

2: Dandelion (Taraxacum officinale): The Immune-Boosting Antibiotic

In the meadows and fields, where most see a humble weed, those in the know recognize a potent healer – Dandelion, a golden harbinger of health. Unveiling its secrets takes us on a journey into the realms of immune-boosting wonders and the extraordinary antibacterial potential of this unassuming plant.

The Golden Healer:
Imagine a field bathed in the golden glow of sunlight, dotted with delicate Dandelion blooms. Beyond their visual charm lies a powerhouse of wellness. Dandelion, often dismissed as a garden nuisance, holds within its roots, leaves, and blossoms a treasure trove of immune-boosting properties, making it an unexpected but extraordinary antibiotic.

The Symphony of Immunity:
Dandelion orchestrates a symphony within your immune system. Rich in vitamins A and C, along with potent antioxidants, it acts as a conductor, harmonizing the body's defense mechanisms. Studies have shown that Dandelion not only enhances the immune response but also exhibits antibacterial effects against various pathogens.

Harvesting the Healing Bounty:
To truly appreciate Dandelion's healing prowess, one must delve into the heart of its medicinal bounty. The leaves, rich in vitamins and minerals, infuse your body with immune-strengthening nutrients. The roots, known for their bitter notes, stimulate digestion and support

liver health, further fortifying your body's natural defenses.

Practical Tips for Embracing Dandelion:

1. Sip on Dandelion Tea:
Replace your regular tea with a soothing cup of Dandelion tea. Harvest the leaves, dry them, and brew a fragrant infusion. This simple ritual not only warms your spirit but also provides a daily dose of immune-boosting goodness.

2. Nutrient-packed Salads:
Embrace Dandelion leaves in your salads. Their slightly bitter taste adds a unique flavor profile, while the nutrients contribute to a resilient immune system. Combine with other greens for a delicious and healthful dish.

3. Dandelion Tinctures:
Explore the world of Dandelion tinctures. Infuse the roots in alcohol or vinegar to create a potent elixir. A few drops daily may just be the immune-boosting tonic your body craves.

4. Leafy Green Smoothies:
Incorporate Dandelion leaves into your morning smoothies. Blending them with fruits masks the bitter taste while retaining the immune-enhancing benefits.

5. Dandelion Infused Oil:
Create a Dandelion-infused oil for topical use. The antimicrobial properties of this oil make it a soothing

addition to your skin-care routine, offering both protection and nourishment.

Reflection Questions:
1. Have you ever overlooked the health potential of common weeds like Dandelion? Why do you think certain plants are dismissed as nuisances?
2. How do you currently support your immune system, and are you open to incorporating unconventional remedies like Dandelion into your routine?
3. What emotions or memories does the image of a golden field of Dandelions evoke for you? How might these emotions influence your perception of this plant as a healing remedy?
4. In what ways can you creatively include Dandelion in your daily meals or rituals? How might this integration impact your overall well-being?
5. Consider the concept of resilience in nature, where even a seemingly fragile flower like Dandelion can thrive. How might adopting a similar resilience mindset benefit your health journey?

Closing Thoughts:
As we conclude our exploration of Dandelion, let its golden presence linger in your mind. In the simplicity of its blossoms lies a profound message – the capacity to flourish even in the face of adversity. Embrace the golden healer, and let Dandelion become a radiant ally in your journey towards a robust and resilient immune system.

Sources:
1. Jeon, H. J., Kang, H. J., Jung, H. J., Kang, Y. S., Lim, C. J., Kim, Y. M., ... Kim, E. H. (2008). Anti-inflammatory

activity of Taraxacum officinale. Journal of Ethnopharmacology, 115(1), 82–88.

2. Hu, C., Kitts, D. D., & Yuan, Y. V. (2005). Antioxidant activities of the flaxseed lignan secoisolariciresinol diglucoside, its aglycone secoisolariciresinol and the mammalian lignans enterodiol and enterolactone in vitro. Food and Chemical Toxicology, 43(5), 753–759.

3. Schütz, K., Carle, R., & Schieber, A. (2006). Taraxacum—a review on its phytochemical and pharmacological profile. Journal of Ethnopharmacology, 107(3), 313–323.

3: Nettle (Urtica dioica): The Antimicrobial and Anti-inflammatory Herb

In the world of herbal remedies, Nettle emerges as a superhero, donning a vibrant green cape and wielding the power to combat microbes and soothe inflammation. This chapter unfolds the extraordinary tale of Nettle (Urtica dioica), a plant that transforms from an ordinary weed to an extraordinary healer, armed with antimicrobial might and anti-inflammatory magic.

The Nettle Chronicles:
Imagine wandering through a sun-dappled forest, your eyes catching a glimpse of lush greenery. Amidst the foliage, Nettle stands tall, a botanical warrior awaiting discovery. In folklore, this herbaceous hero has been known for centuries as a guardian of health, with tales of its remarkable powers echoing through the ages.

The Nettle Arsenal:
Nettle, with its serrated leaves and stinging hairs, might seem like an unlikely ally. However, within this seemingly prickly exterior lies a botanical arsenal ready to combat microbes and alleviate inflammation. Rich in vitamins, minerals, and bioactive compounds, Nettle's prowess extends beyond the garden to offer a holistic approach to wellness.

Antimicrobial Marvel:
Picture this: Nettle standing as a sentinel, repelling harmful microbes with its natural defense mechanisms. Studies have shown that extracts from Nettle possess antimicrobial properties, making it a formidable

opponent against various bacteria and fungi. This unassuming herb transforms into a microbial superhero, protecting your body from unseen invaders.

Practical Tips for Harnessing Nettle's Powers:

1. Nettle Infusion for Immunity:
Brew a nourishing nettle infusion by steeping dried leaves in hot water. This herbal elixir, rich in vitamins and minerals, becomes a powerhouse for immune support.

2. Nettle Pesto:
Elevate your culinary adventures with a Nettle pesto. Blending fresh Nettle leaves with garlic, nuts, and olive oil creates a delicious spread rich in anti-inflammatory and antimicrobial goodness.

3. Topical Nettle Poultice:
Craft a soothing poultice by blending fresh Nettle leaves and applying the mixture topically. This DIY remedy can help alleviate inflammation associated with skin conditions or joint discomfort.

4. Nettle Tea for Allergies:
Combat seasonal allergies with a cup of Nettle tea. Its natural antihistamine properties may offer relief from common allergy symptoms, providing a botanical alternative to over-the-counter medications.

5. Nettle Hair Rinse:
Enhance your hair care routine with a Nettle-infused hair rinse. Boil Nettle leaves, let the concoction cool,

and use it as a final hair rinse. The antimicrobial properties may contribute to a healthier scalp.

Reflection Questions:
1. Consider the concept of "stinging" Nettle. How might challenges or discomfort in life parallel the initial sting of this herb, only to reveal transformative healing benefits?
2. Reflect on your current approach to immune support. How open are you to incorporating unconventional remedies like Nettle into your routine? What factors influence your willingness to explore alternative therapies?
3. Imagine your kitchen as an apothecary. How might you creatively integrate Nettle into your daily meals to maximize its antimicrobial and anti-inflammatory benefits?
4. In what ways can you adopt Nettle as a holistic remedy, not just for physical ailments but also for soothing mental or emotional inflammation?
5. Reflect on the multifaceted nature of Nettle, offering both defensive and nurturing qualities. How might embodying a similar duality benefit your approach to well-being?

Closing Thoughts:
As we close the chapter on Nettle, let the vibrant green leaves linger in your imagination. Nettle, with its antimicrobial valor and anti-inflammatory charm, beckons you to explore the richness of nature's pharmacy. Embrace this botanical hero, let it infuse vitality into your life, and allow Nettle to become a trusted companion on your journey to vibrant well-being.

Sources:

1. Mittman, P. (1990). Randomized, double-blind study of freeze-dried Urtica dioica in the treatment of allergic rhinitis. Planta Medica, 56(01), 44–47.
2. Roschek, B., Fink, R. C., McMichael, M., Alberte, R. S., & Alberte, R. S. (2009). Nettle extract (Urtica dioica) affects key receptors and enzymes associated with allergic rhinitis. Phytotherapy Research, 23(7), 920–926.
3. Dastmalchi, K., Damien Dorman, H. J., & Oinonen, P. P. (2008). Chemical composition and in vitro antioxidative activity of a lemon balm (Melissa officinalis L.) extract. LWT - Food Science and Technology, 41(3), 391–400.

4: Milk Thistle (Silybum marianum): A Potent Antimicrobial Adventure

In the lush tapestry of herbal wonders, there's a spiky guardian that goes beyond its thorny exterior to unveil a remarkable secret – Milk Thistle, the unsung hero in the world of potent antimicrobials. Join me on an exciting adventure into the realm of Silybum marianum, where spikes give way to healing might, and every twist and turn reveals a new facet of this botanical superhero.

The Thistle's Secret Arsenal:
Imagine a medieval garden guarded by Milk Thistle, its regal purple flowers standing tall against the breeze. Within this fortress, Milk Thistle unveils its secret arsenal – a compound known as silymarin. This unassuming thistle, often overlooked in gardens, transforms into a formidable defender against microbial invaders.

Silymarin: Nature's Shield:
Silymarin, the unsung hero of Milk Thistle, emerges as a natural shield against microbes. Studies have shown that this compound possesses potent antimicrobial properties, making Milk Thistle a robust ally in the battle against bacterial and fungal foes. Imagine silymarin as a guardian knight, protecting your body's citadel from unseen invaders.

Practical Tips for Welcoming Milk Thistle:

1. Milk Thistle Tea Ritual:
Begin your Milk Thistle adventure with a soothing tea ritual. Steep Milk Thistle seeds in hot water for a fragrant infusion. This botanical brew becomes your daily elixir, infusing your system with silymarin's protective embrace.

2. Silymarin Super Salad:
Elevate your culinary escapades with a Silymarin Super Salad. Toasted Milk Thistle seeds sprinkled over fresh greens not only add a delightful crunch but also imbue your meal with antimicrobial prowess.

3. DIY Milk Thistle Tincture:
Embark on a DIY project and create your Milk Thistle tincture. Soak crushed Milk Thistle seeds in alcohol, let time work its magic, and voilà – you have a potent elixir at your disposal. A few drops daily can become your herbal shield.

4. Milk Thistle Capsules:
If culinary adventures aren't your forte, opt for Milk Thistle capsules. Convenient and packed with silymarin, these capsules offer a hassle-free way to integrate this botanical defender into your daily routine.

5. Milk Thistle Skin Salve:
Extend Milk Thistle's protection to your skin. Infuse Milk Thistle oil with your favorite carrier oil, creating a skin salve that not only moisturizes but also shields against microbial mischief.

Just for fun, and to help you remember the things you have learned about Milk Thistle, here are 5 Quizzes for you:

Quiz 1: Silymarin Showdown
1. What is the active compound in Milk Thistle responsible for its antimicrobial properties?
   a. Thistlelicious
   b. Silymarin
   c. Marianumagic

Quiz 2: Milk Thistle Mythbuster
2. True or False: Milk Thistle is only beneficial for liver health and doesn't have antimicrobial properties.

Quiz 3: Herbal Guardians
3. Which metaphor best describes Milk Thistle's role against microbes?
   a. Guardian Knight
   b. Secret Spy
   c. Happy Gardener

Quiz 4: DIY Adventure
4. What is one DIY project mentioned to incorporate Milk Thistle into your routine?
   a. Bungee Jumping with Thistles
   b. Milk Thistle Tincture
   c. Thistle Artistry Class

Quiz 5: Culinary Exploration
5. How can you add Milk Thistle to your culinary repertoire?
   a. Turn it into a Milkshake
   b. Sprinkle seeds on a salad

c. Wear it as a hat

Reflection Questions:

1. Consider the image of Milk Thistle as a botanical knight. How might this metaphor influence your perception of its role in your health journey?
2. Reflect on your current understanding of herbal remedies. How open are you to exploring lesser-known plants like Milk Thistle for their antimicrobial benefits?
3. Imagine incorporating Milk Thistle into your daily routine. How might this botanical adventure impact your overall well-being, and what changes are you willing to make?
4. Milk Thistle's thorny appearance contrasts with its healing properties. How might this juxtaposition resonate with experiences in your own life, where challenges led to unexpected growth or strength?
5. Think about Milk Thistle as your herbal ally. How can you create a ritual around its use to make it a delightful and sustainable part of your daily life?

Closing Thoughts:
As we close the chapter on Milk Thistle, envision the thorny guardian standing tall in your metaphorical garden of well-being. Embrace the spikes, savor the silymarin, and let Milk Thistle be your guide in this enchanting adventure into the realm of potent antimicrobials.

Sources:
1. Abenavoli, L., Capasso, R., Milic, N., & Capasso, F. (2018). Milk thistle in liver diseases: Past, present, future. Phytotherapy Research, 32(11), 2202–2213.

2. Rainone, F. (2005). Milk thistle. American Family Physician, 72(7), 1285–1288.

25

5: Cat's Claw (Uncaria tomentosa): An Immune-Boosting Antimicrobial Marvel

In the heart of the rainforest, where vibrant life dances to the rhythm of nature, a secret lies in the tangle of vines. Cat's Claw, the mystical guardian of the jungle, emerges as an extraordinary immune-boosting antimicrobial marvel. This chapter unravels the tale of Uncaria tomentosa, where the wild and the healing collide, offering you a passport to an untamed world of well-being.

Jungle Symphony of Healing:
Close your eyes and let your imagination roam through the lush canopy of the Amazon rainforest. Amidst the cacophony of exotic sounds, Cat's Claw stands tall. Its twisted vines, resembling a cat's claws, hold within them the promise of immune-boosting magic. Welcome to the jungle symphony of healing, where Cat's Claw takes center stage.

Uncaria tomentosa: The Jungle's Gift to You:
Cat's Claw isn't just a vine; it's a botanical gift from the jungle. Rich in compounds like oxindole alkaloids and quinovic acid glycosides, Cat's Claw becomes your ally in the quest for a resilient immune system. Imagine it as a guardian, patrolling your body's defenses and ensuring harmony within.

Antimicrobial Adventure:
Embark on an antimicrobial adventure as Cat's Claw unleashes its potency. Studies reveal that this jungle marvel possesses antimicrobial properties, making it a formidable force against bacteria, viruses, and fungi.

Picture it as a jungle warrior, equipped to defend your health on multiple fronts.

Practical Tips for Embracing Cat's Claw:

1. Cat's Claw Tincture Ritual:
Start your Cat's Claw journey with a daily tincture ritual. A few drops under the tongue can be your secret weapon against microbial invaders, offering your immune system an empowering boost.

2. Cat's Claw Tea Ceremony:
Craft a soothing Cat's Claw tea ceremony. Steep the bark in hot water, allowing the essence of the jungle to infuse into your cup. This aromatic elixir becomes a daily celebration of immune-boosting vitality.

3. Smoothie Jungle Blend:
Transform your morning smoothie into a jungle blend. Mix Cat's Claw powder with tropical fruits for a delicious, immune-boosting concoction. Your taste buds will dance to the rhythm of the rainforest.

4. Cat's Claw Capsules Expedition:
Opt for the convenience of Cat's Claw capsules. These capsules, filled with the potency of the jungle, become your daily expedition into the world of immune resilience.

5. Cat's Claw Topical Magic:
Unleash Cat's Claw's magic on your skin. Create a topical salve by infusing Cat's Claw with a carrier oil. This jungle balm not only soothes but also provides an extra layer of protection against microbial intruders.

To help you with ideas of enhancing Cat's Claw for yourself and friends and community I have put together some actions below for you to do.

Useful Actions:

Action 1: Wild Wellness Pledge
Take a moment to pledge allegiance to your wellness. Commit to exploring the wild side of well-being with Cat's Claw as your jungle companion.

Action 2: Daily Cat's Claw Challenge
Challenge yourself to incorporate Cat's Claw into your daily routine for the next 30 days. Notice and document the changes in your energy, mood, and overall health.

Action 3: Jungle Blend Smoothie Contest
Share your most creative Cat's Claw smoothie recipe on social media. Tag friends to join the jungle blend movement and create a ripple effect of wellness inspiration.

Action 4: Cat's Claw Tea Time Gathering
Host a Cat's Claw tea time gathering with friends or family. Share the immune-boosting magic and make it a joyful celebration of health and togetherness.

Action 5: Gift the Jungle
Gift Cat's Claw to a friend or loved one. Spread the jungle's healing touch by sharing the knowledge and power of this botanical marvel.

Closing Thoughts:
As we conclude this chapter, envision Cat's Claw as your ticket to the heart of the jungle, where resilience and vitality thrive. Let the wild essence of Uncaria tomentosa infuse into your life, empowering your immune system and becoming the untamed ally you never knew you needed.

Sources:

1. Sandoval, M., Charbonnet, R. M., Okuhama, N. N., Roberts, J., Krenova, Z., Trentacosti, A. M., ... Miller, M. J. (2002). Cat's Claw inhibits TNFα production and scavenges free radicals: Role in cytoprotection. Free Radical Biology and Medicine, 29(1), 71–78.
2. Keplinger, K., Laus, G., Wurm, M., Dierich, M. P., & Teppner, H. (1999). Uncaria tomentosa (Willd.) DC.—ethnomedicinal use and new pharmacological, toxicological and botanical results. Journal of Ethnopharmacology, 64(1), 23–34.

6: Astragalus (Astragalus membranaceus): The Immune-Stimulator Extravaganza

In the grand theater of wellness, imagine a star taking the center stage, radiating vitality and resilience. That star is Astragalus, a botanical virtuoso in the symphony of immune health. This chapter unveils the captivating tale of Astragalus membranaceus, a herbal maestro conducting a spectacular immune-stimulating performance that promises to transform your well-being into a harmonious masterpiece.

The Rise of Astragalus:
Picture yourself in an ancient apothecary, surrounded by jars of mystical herbs. Astragalus emerges as the crown jewel, a revered tonic celebrated for centuries. Today, this herbal virtuoso steps into the limelight, ready to compose a melody of immune-stimulating brilliance in the concert of your health.

Astragalus: The Immune Composer:
Astragalus is not just an herb; it's a symphony conductor orchestrating immune harmony. Rich in polysaccharides, flavonoids, and saponins, Astragalus becomes the virtuoso leading the immune system in a crescendo of strength. Imagine it as a guardian angel, nurturing and fortifying your body's defenses.

Immune-Stimulating Serenade:
Close your eyes and listen to the serenade of Astragalus as it stimulates your immune system. Studies have shown that the compounds within this herb not only activate immune cells but also enhance their ability to combat invaders. Astragalus becomes a musical

crescendo, empowering your body's defenses to play a protective melody.

Practical Tips for Integrating Astragalus Magic:

1. Astragalus Elixir Sunrise:
Start your day with an Astragalus elixir. Mix Astragalus root slices with hot water, honey, and a splash of lemon. This golden concoction becomes your sunrise ritual, infusing your morning with immune-stimulating magic.

2. Astragalus Broth Bonanza:
Elevate your culinary skills with an Astragalus broth. Simmer Astragalus root with vegetables and spices to create a hearty, immune-boosting elixir. Let the aroma fill your kitchen as you savor the healthful delights.

3. Astragalus Tea Party:
Host an Astragalus tea party with friends. Steep Astragalus root slices in hot water, creating a fragrant tea. This social gathering not only warms your heart but also fortifies your immune camaraderie.

4. Astragalus Smoothie Symphony:
Infuse your smoothie routine with Astragalus. Blend Astragalus powder with berries, spinach, and a dollop of yogurt for a delicious immune-stimulating symphony. Let the vibrant colors and flavors dance on your palate.

5. Astragalus Tincture Toast:
Craft an Astragalus tincture to elevate your wellness toast. Soak Astragalus root in alcohol, creating a potent elixir. A daily toast with a few drops of this tincture becomes a celebration of health and vitality.

The Life-Changing Impact:

Imagine a life where your immune system is not just functioning but thriving. Astragalus opens the door to this possibility, inviting you into a world where your body is an impenetrable fortress against common ailments. The impact of incorporating Astragalus into your routine is nothing short of transformative.

Actionable Advice:

1. Daily Dose of Astragalus Love:
Integrate Astragalus into your daily routine. Whether through elixirs, teas, or tinctures, make it a daily commitment to give your immune system the love and support it deserves.

2. Share the Melody:
Spread the word about Astragalus. Share your favorite recipes and immune-stimulating experiences with friends and family. The more we harmonize our health practices, the stronger our collective well-being becomes.

3. Celebrate Small Wins:
Acknowledge and celebrate the small wins on your wellness journey. Whether it's completing a week of Astragalus-infused mornings or trying a new recipe, every step counts toward a healthier you.

4. Create Rituals of Wellness:
Turn your Astragalus routines into wellness rituals. Find joy in the process, savor the flavors, and appreciate the

positive impact on your health. Wellness is not just a destination; it's a journey to be relished.

5. Listen to Your Body's Symphony:
Pay attention to the symphony within. Notice how your body responds to the immune-stimulating magic of Astragalus. Whether it's increased energy, better sleep, or a general sense of well-being, let your body's melody guide you.

Closing Harmony:
As we draw the curtain on this chapter, envision a life where your immune system performs a harmonious melody, and Astragalus is the conductor guiding every note. Let this herbal maestro be the key to unlocking a new chapter of well-being, where vitality, resilience, and health become the crescendo of your life's symphony.

Sources:
1. Block, K. I., Mead, M. N., & Zhang, X. (2009). Immune system effects of echinacea, ginseng, and astragalus: a review. Integrative Cancer Therapies, 8(3), 208–227.
2. Shao, B. M., Xu, W., Dai, H., Tu, P., & Li, Z. (2004). Gao, X. M. - A study on the immune receptors for polysaccharides from the roots of Astragalus membranaceus, a Chinese medicinal herb. Biochemical and Biophysical Research Communications, 320(4), 1103–1111.

7: Oregano Oil (Origanum vulgare): The Strong Antibacterial and Antiviral Marvel

Welcome to the aromatic world of Oregano Oil, where the essence of Origanum vulgare transforms into a potent defender against bacterial and viral intruders. This chapter unfolds the captivating tale of a culinary herb that takes on a new role as a powerful antibacterial and antiviral superhero, ready to invigorate your health journey.

Oregano Unleashed:
Picture a Mediterranean kitchen, where the scent of fresh herbs fills the air. In this aromatic symphony, Oregano Oil emerges as a hero, not just enhancing flavors but also combating unseen foes. This chapter invites you to explore the untapped potential of Oregano, a culinary delight turned antibacterial and antiviral marvel.

Oregano Oil: The Mighty Defender:
Oregano Oil isn't just a condiment; it's a robust defender armed with antibacterial and antiviral weapons. Rich in compounds like carvacrol and thymol, Oregano Oil becomes your ally in the battle against microbial invaders. Imagine it as a fearless knight, standing guard to protect your well-being.

Antibacterial Ballet, Antiviral Symphony:
Envision Oregano Oil as a performer on a microbial stage, engaging in a delicate ballet against bacteria and orchestrating a symphony to combat viruses. Scientific studies reveal that the potent compounds in Oregano Oil exhibit both antibacterial and antiviral effects, making it a versatile and holistic addition to your health arsenal.

Practical Tips for Harnessing Oregano's Magic:

1. Oregano Oil Inhalation Ritual:
Kickstart your day with an Oregano Oil inhalation ritual. Add a few drops to hot water, cover your head with a towel, and inhale deeply. This invigorating practice not only clears your respiratory passages but also infuses your day with antibacterial freshness.

2. Immune-Boosting Oregano Tea:
Brew a cup of immune-boosting Oregano tea. Steep fresh or dried Oregano leaves in hot water, adding a dash of honey. This herbal infusion becomes a comforting ally, supporting your immune system against viral invaders.

3. Oregano Oil Salad Dressing Delight:
Elevate your salads with an Oregano Oil dressing. Mix Oregano Oil with olive oil, garlic, and a hint of lemon. This not only adds a burst of flavor to your greens but also introduces antibacterial elements to your meal.

4. Antiviral Oregano Oil Foot Soak:
Treat your feet to an antiviral Oregano Oil foot soak. Add a few drops to warm water, allowing the soothing and invigorating properties to work their magic. This simple ritual not only relaxes your feet but also contributes to overall well-being.

5. Oregano Oil Respiratory Steam Show:
Create an Oregano Oil respiratory steam show. Add a few drops to a bowl of hot water, cover your head, and inhale deeply. This therapeutic steam not

only supports respiratory health but also acts as an antibacterial and antiviral spa for your senses.

Reflection Questions:

1. Reflect on your current health routine. How open are you to incorporating unconventional remedies like Oregano Oil into your daily practices for antibacterial and antiviral support?
2. Consider the aromatic symphony of Oregano Oil. How does its scent and flavor enhance your culinary experiences, and how might this impact your overall well-being?
3. Imagine Oregano Oil as a fearless knight in your health journey. How might adopting a similar resilience mindset positively affect your approach to well-being?
4. Think about the delicate ballet and symphony of antibacterial and antiviral effects. In what ways can you envision Oregano Oil supporting your immune system against microbial invaders?
5. Reflect on your feelings after trying one of the Oregano Oil rituals or recipes. How did the experience impact your mood, energy levels, or sense of well-being?

The Life-Changing Impact:

Embracing Oregano Oil isn't just a culinary adventure; it's a transformative journey toward a healthier, more resilient you. The impact of incorporating Oregano Oil into your routine extends beyond antibacterial and antiviral support; it's about invigorating your senses and elevating your well-being.

Actionable Advice:

1. Oregano Oil Challenge:
Challenge yourself to a 30-day Oregano Oil adventure. Experiment with different rituals and recipes, and document the changes in your well-being. Share your journey with friends and inspire a collective commitment to health.

2. Oregano Oil Wellness Journal:
Create an Oregano Oil wellness journal. Record your experiences, feelings, and any noticeable changes in your health. This journal becomes a personal guide to understanding the impact of Oregano Oil on your well-being.

3. Share the Oregano Magic:
Share your favorite Oregano Oil recipes and rituals with your social circle. Encourage friends and family to join the Oregano movement, fostering a community dedicated to antibacterial and antiviral well-being.

4. Mindful Culinary Exploration:
Approach your culinary adventures with mindfulness. When using Oregano Oil in recipes, savor the aroma, appreciate the flavors, and acknowledge the potential health benefits. Transforming cooking into a mindful experience amplifies the positive impact on well-being.

5. Educate and Empower:
Take the opportunity to educate others about the benefits of Oregano Oil. Empower those around you with knowledge about antibacterial and antiviral

support, and collectively contribute to a community dedicated to holistic wellness.

Closing Notes:

As we conclude this chapter, envision Oregano Oil not just as a kitchen companion but as a steadfast ally in your journey toward vibrant health. Let the aromatic symphony, the delicate ballet, and the fearless knight inspire you to explore the transformative potential of Origanum vulgare in your life.

Sources:
1. Force, M., & Sparks, W. S. (2008). Antifungal effects of volatile compounds generated by essential oils on fungi associated with Achoria grisella (Lepidoptera: Pyralidae). Journal of Economic Entomology, 101(1), 173–183.
2. Nostro, A., Blanco, A. R., Cannatelli, M. A., Enea, V., Flamini, G., Morelli, I., ... & Alonzo, V. (2004). Susceptibility of methicillin-resistant staphylococci to oregano essential oil, carvacrol and thymol. FEMS Microbiology Letters, 230(2), 191–195.

8: Echinacea (Echinacea purpurea): A Powerful Immune Booster Extravaganza

Welcome to the vibrant world of Echinacea, where the petals of Echinacea purpurea unfold into a powerful symphony of immune-boosting wonders. This chapter embarks on a captivating journey through meadows of purple blooms, revealing the secret behind Echinacea's prowess as a robust immune booster that can transform your health narrative.

Petals of Strength:
Imagine a field of Echinacea, each petal holding the promise of resilience and vitality. Echinacea is not just a wildflower; it's a botanical powerhouse that has adorned the wellness routines of many seeking to fortify their immune systems. In this chapter, we delve into the petals of strength, unlocking the potential of Echinacea to uplift your well-being.

Echinacea: Nature's Immune Conductor:
Echinacea isn't just a flower; it's nature's conductor orchestrating a harmony within your immune system. Bursting with bioactive compounds like alkamides, polysaccharides, and flavonoids, Echinacea becomes the maestro leading your body's defense against potential threats. Envision it as the conductor of a grand orchestra, bringing together immune elements in a symphony of strength.

Immune-Boosting Symphony:
Picture your immune system as a symphony waiting to be conducted. Studies suggest that Echinacea can enhance the activity of immune cells, promoting a

robust defense against invading pathogens. Echinacea's symphony is not just a melody; it's a powerful anthem of protection, ready to elevate your well-being.

Practical Tips for Immune Elevation:

1. Echinacea Tincture Sunrise Ritual:
Start your mornings with an Echinacea tincture ritual. A few drops under your tongue become the sunrise notes, awakening your immune symphony. This daily practice instills a sense of readiness to face the day's challenges.

2. Echinacea Tea Celebration:
Brew a cup of Echinacea tea to celebrate your health. Steep Echinacea flowers in hot water, adding a touch of honey. This herbal infusion becomes a moment of reflection and gratitude for the resilience within.

3. Echinacea and Citrus Infused Water Parade:
Join the hydration parade with Echinacea and citrus-infused water. Combine Echinacea tea with slices of citrus fruits for a refreshing elixir that not only quenches your thirst but also fortifies your immune defenses.

4. Echinacea Honey Drizzle Delight:
Elevate your culinary adventures with an Echinacea honey drizzle. Mix Echinacea tincture with raw honey, creating a sweet and immune-boosting delight to enhance your favorite dishes.

5. Echinacea Capsules Support Routine:
Integrate Echinacea capsules into your daily routine. This convenient form of Echinacea allows you to

effortlessly incorporate its immune-boosting benefits into your life, supporting your well-being on the go.

Reflection Questions:

1. Reflect on your current approach to immune health. How open are you to exploring botanical allies like Echinacea to enhance your immune symphony?
2. Consider the concept of your immune system as a symphony. How might visualizing this intricate interplay influence your perception of well-being and your body's natural defense mechanisms?
3. Envision Echinacea as the conductor of your immune orchestra. In what ways can you actively contribute to this symphony, fostering a harmonious relationship between your lifestyle and immune health?
4. Think about the moments of ritual and celebration involving Echinacea. How might incorporating these practices into your daily life influence your overall mindset and well-being?
5. Reflect on the bioactive compounds in Echinacea. How does this knowledge empower you to make informed decisions about incorporating Echinacea into your wellness routine?

Case Studies:

Case Study 1: Sarah's Winter Wellness Journey:
Meet Sarah, a busy professional navigating the challenges of a hectic winter season. Struggling with seasonal health concerns, she decided to embark on a winter wellness journey with Echinacea. By incorporating Echinacea tea and tinctures into her routine, Sarah noticed a significant improvement in her

overall well-being. The immune-boosting properties of Echinacea became her secret weapon against winter blues, empowering her to face each day with vitality.

Case Study 2: Mike's Travel Companion:
Mike, a frequent traveler exposed to various environments, faced immune challenges due to his on-the-go lifestyle. Seeking a natural solution, he discovered the convenience of Echinacea capsules. Incorporating them into his travel routine, Mike found that Echinacea became his reliable companion, providing immune support and helping him stay resilient during his adventures.

Case Study 3: Maria's Hydration Journey:
Maria, a fitness enthusiast, wanted to enhance her hydration routine with immune-boosting elements. Inspired by Echinacea's benefits, she experimented with Echinacea and citrus-infused water. Not only did this delightful concoction elevate her hydration game, but it also became a symbolic celebration of her commitment to overall well-being.

The Life-Changing Impact:

Echinacea isn't just a botanical remedy; it's a transformative force that can positively impact your life. The life-changing impact of incorporating Echinacea into your routine extends beyond immune support; it's about embracing resilience, celebrating well-being, and nurturing the symphony within.

Actionable Advice:

1. Echinacea Immune Challenge:
Challenge yourself to a 30-day Echinacea immune challenge. Experiment with different Echinacea rituals and note any changes in your energy levels, mood, or overall well-being. Share your journey with friends and encourage them to join the challenge.

2. Gratitude Reflection Practice:
Incorporate a daily reflection practice expressing gratitude to the creator for your immune system and overall well-being. Use this moment of reflection to acknowledge the strength within and the support Echinacea provides.

3. Create Immune Celebration Rituals:
Establish immune celebration rituals involving Echinacea. Whether it's a morning tincture ritual or an evening tea ceremony, infuse these moments with intention and celebration of your body's resilience.

4. Educate Your Wellness Circle:
Share your Echinacea journey with friends and family. Educate them about the benefits of Echinacea and encourage them to explore its immune-boosting potential. Create a supportive wellness circle dedicated to thriving together.

5. Listen to Your Immune Symphony:
Pay attention to the symphony within. Notice how incorporating Echinacea into your routine influences your overall well-being. Listen to the subtle notes of

resilience and strength, and let your immune symphony guide you toward a healthier and more vibrant life.

Closing Harmony:

As we conclude this chapter, envision Echinacea not just as a flower in the field but as a powerful conductor leading your immune symphony. Let the petals of strength inspire you to embrace resilience, celebrate well-being, and nurture the transformative potential of Echinacea in your life.

Sources:

1. Shah, S. A., Sander, S., White, C. M., Rinaldi, M., & Coleman, C. I. (2007). Evaluation of echinacea for the prevention and treatment of the common cold: a meta-analysis. The Lancet Infectious Diseases, 7(7), 473–480.
2. Schoop, R., Klein, P., & Suter, A. (2006). Echinacea in the prevention of induced rhinovirus colds: a meta-analysis. Clinical Therapeutics, 28(2), 174–183.
3. Barrett, B. (2003). Medicinal properties of Echinacea: a critical review. Phytomedicine, 10(1), 66–86.

9: Goldenseal (Hydrastis canadensis): An Antibacterial and Immune-Booster Adventure

Step into the world of Goldenseal, where the golden roots of Hydrastis canadensis weave a tapestry of antibacterial wonders and immune-boosting magic. This chapter invites you on a captivating adventure through the lush woodlands where Goldenseal flourishes, unlocking the secrets that make it a botanical hero in the realm of well-being.

Golden Roots, Golden Resilience:
Imagine a forest clearing, bathed in golden hues, where the roots of Goldenseal delve deep into the earth, absorbing the vitality of the land. Goldenseal is not just a herb; it's a treasure trove of antibacterial properties and immune-boosting prowess. Join us as we unravel the golden resilience of Hydrastis canadensis.

Goldenseal: Nature's Antibacterial Artisan:
Goldenseal isn't just a herb; it's nature's artisan crafting antibacterial masterpieces. Enriched with berberine, hydrastine, and canadine, Goldenseal becomes the brushstroke painting a canvas of defense against bacterial intruders. Visualize it as the artist sculpting a shield of protection around your well-being.

Immune-Boosting Symphony:
Picture your immune system as a symphony echoing through the body. Studies suggest that Goldenseal, with its antibacterial properties, can enhance the immune system's ability to orchestrate a harmonious defense. Goldenseal's symphony is not just a melody; it's a robust anthem of vitality ready to elevate your health.

Practical Tips for Goldenseal Empowerment:

1. Golden Elixir Morning Ritual:
Begin your mornings with a Golden Elixir ritual. Mix a few drops of Goldenseal tincture with warm water, creating a golden elixir that kickstarts your day with antibacterial and immune-boosting energy.

2. Goldenseal Infused Honey Magic:
Transform your honey jar into a powerhouse with Goldenseal. Mix Goldenseal powder into raw honey, creating a delicious and immune-boosting treat to accompany your morning toast or evening tea.

3. Golden Tea Ceremony:
Host a Golden Tea ceremony with friends or family. Steep Goldenseal root in hot water, creating a fragrant and antibacterial-infused tea. This social gathering becomes a celebration of well-being and resilience.

4. Goldenseal Respiratory Steam Retreat:
Treat yourself to a Goldenseal respiratory steam retreat. Add Goldenseal root to hot water, cover your head, and inhale deeply. This therapeutic steam not only supports respiratory health but also introduces antibacterial elements to your self-care routine.

5. Goldenseal Capsules Daily Shield:
Incorporate Goldenseal capsules into your daily routine. These capsules, filled with the golden essence of Hydrastis canadensis, become your daily shield against bacterial challenges, empowering your immune system.

Reflection Questions:

1. Reflect on your current knowledge of antibacterial and immune-boosting herbs. How open are you to exploring the golden realms of Goldenseal to enhance your well-being?
2. Consider Goldenseal as nature's artisan. How might visualizing Goldenseal's antibacterial properties influence your perception of its role in supporting your health?
3. Envision your immune system as a symphony. In what ways can you actively contribute to this symphony, fostering a harmonious relationship between your lifestyle and immune health?
4. Reflect on the practical tips for Goldenseal empowerment. How might incorporating these rituals and recipes into your daily life positively impact your well-being?
5. Think about the golden resilience of Goldenseal. How does the knowledge of its antibacterial and immune-boosting properties empower you to take charge of your health journey?

Case Studies:

Case Study 1: Emily's Winter Wellness Guardian:
Meet Emily, a teacher navigating the challenges of winter in a bustling school environment. Concerned about seasonal health issues, she incorporated Goldenseal capsules into her daily routine. Over the winter months, Emily noticed a significant reduction in the frequency of common ailments, attributing her resilience to the antibacterial and immune-boosting support of Goldenseal.

Case Study 2: James' Respiratory Retreat:
James, an avid hiker, faced occasional respiratory challenges due to his outdoor adventures. Seeking a natural solution, he introduced Goldenseal respiratory steams into his post-hike self-care routine. Not only did this ritual provide relief to his respiratory system, but it also became a golden retreat, enhancing his overall well-being.

Case Study 3: Sarah's Golden Tea Celebrations:
Sarah, a wellness enthusiast, embraced Goldenseal as part of her daily rituals. Hosting Golden Tea celebrations with friends, she found joy in sharing the antibacterial and immune-boosting magic of Goldenseal. These gatherings became not only a celebration of well-being but also an opportunity to educate and inspire her social circle.

Case Study 4: Michael's Golden Honey Mastery:
Michael, a culinary artist, explored the world of herbal infusions in his kitchen. Intrigued by Goldenseal's antibacterial properties, he mastered the art of infusing raw honey with Goldenseal powder. This Golden Honey creation not only elevated the flavors of his dishes but also became a culinary masterpiece infused with immune-boosting magic.

The Life-Changing Impact:

Goldenseal isn't just a herb; it's a life-changing force that can positively impact your well-being. The golden resilience of Hydrastis canadensis extends beyond antibacterial support; it's about embracing vitality, celebrating health, and nurturing the transformative potential of Goldenseal in your life.

Actionable Advice:

1. Golden Wellness Journal:
Create a Golden Wellness journal. Document your experiences, feelings, and any noticeable changes in your health as you incorporate Goldenseal into your routine. This journal becomes a personal guide on your journey to well-being.

2. Share the Goldenseal Magic:
Share your experiences with Goldenseal with friends and family. Educate them about the benefits of this antibacterial and immune-boosting herb. Encourage your social circle to explore the golden realms of Goldenseal together.

3. Golden Elixir Challenge:
Challenge yourself to a 30-day Golden Elixir adventure. Experiment with different Goldenseal rituals and recipes, and observe how these practices positively impact your energy levels, mood, or overall well-being. Encourage friends to embark on the challenge with you.

4. Golden Rituals of Celebration:
Establish Golden Rituals of Celebration involving Goldenseal. Whether it's a morning elixir or an evening tea ceremony, infuse these moments with intention and celebrate the golden resilience within.

5. Listen to Your

Golden Symphony:
Pay attention to the golden symphony within. Notice how incorporating Goldenseal into your routine influences your overall well-being. Listen to the subtle notes of resilience and strength, and let your golden symphony guide you toward a healthier and more vibrant life.

Closing Harmony:

As we conclude this chapter, envision Goldenseal not just as a herb in the forest but as a golden guardian of your well-being. Let the golden roots, golden rituals, and golden resilience inspire you to embrace vitality, celebrate health, and nurture the transformative potential of Hydrastis canadensis in your life.

Sources:

1. Melchart, D., Walther, E., Linde, K., Brandmaier, R., Lersch, C., & Echinacea, B. (1998). Echinacea root extracts for the prevention of upper respiratory tract infections: a double-blind, placebo-controlled randomized trial. Archives of Family Medicine, 7(6), 541–545.
2. Cernakova, M., Kost'alova, D., & Kettmann, V. (2002). Isolation and characterization of alkamides from Rudbeckia fulgida. Planta Medica, 68(5), 408–413.
3. Hussain, H., Hussain, J., Al-Harrasi, A., & Green, I. R. (2011). Chemistry and biology of the genus Hydrastis. Chemistry & Biodiversity, 8(4), 668–681.

10: Ginger (Zingiber officinale): An Antimicrobial Immune System Supporter

Welcome to the zesty realm of Ginger, where the rhizomes of Zingiber officinale unfold as a powerhouse of antimicrobial wonders and immune-boosting magic. In this chapter, we embark on a journey through the aromatic landscapes where Ginger thrives, unraveling the secrets that make it a versatile ally in fortifying your immune system and elevating your overall well-being.

Zest for Life, Zest for Health:
Imagine a kitchen filled with the warm and invigorating aroma of fresh Ginger. Ginger is not just a spice; it's a burst of flavor that carries the essence of health. Join us as we explore the zest for life that Ginger brings and how it can be your secret weapon in supporting a robust immune system.

Ginger: Nature's Antimicrobial Maestro:
Ginger isn't just a spice; it's nature's maestro orchestrating antimicrobial symphonies. Enriched with compounds like gingerol and shogaol, Ginger becomes the virtuoso playing a melody of defense against microbial intruders. Visualize it as the conductor leading your immune orchestra to new heights.

Immune-Boosting Symphony:
Picture your immune system as a symphony awaiting the conductor's cue. Studies suggest that Ginger, with its antimicrobial properties, can enhance the immune system's ability to orchestrate a harmonious defense. Ginger's symphony is not just a melody; it's a powerful anthem of vitality ready to elevate your health.

Practical Tips for Gingerful Wellness:

1. Morning Ginger Zing Elixir:
Start your mornings with a Ginger Zing Elixir. Mix freshly grated Ginger with hot water, a dash of lemon, and honey. This zesty elixir becomes a wake-up call for your immune system, infusing your day with energy and antimicrobial support.

2. Ginger Spice Tea Ceremony:
Host a Ginger Spice Tea ceremony with friends or family. Steep fresh Ginger slices, cinnamon, and cloves in hot water, creating a fragrant and immune-boosting tea. This social gathering becomes a celebration of well-being and a moment to savor the warmth of health.

3. Ginger Turmeric Golden Milk Delight:
Elevate your evenings with a Ginger Turmeric Golden Milk Delight. Blend fresh Ginger, turmeric, and a pinch of black pepper with warm milk. This golden elixir not only soothes your senses but also introduces powerful antimicrobial and immune-supporting elements to your routine.

4. Ginger Lemon Honey Wellness Shot:
Integrate a Ginger Lemon Honey Wellness Shot into your daily routine. Blend Ginger juice, lemon juice, and a spoonful of raw honey. This potent shot becomes a quick and effective way to kickstart your immune system and infuse your day with Gingerful wellness.

5. Ginger-infused Culinary Adventures:
Embark on Ginger-infused culinary adventures. Incorporate fresh or powdered Ginger into your favorite dishes, soups, and salads. Transforming your meals into Gingerful delights not only enhances flavor but also introduces antimicrobial support to your diet.

Reflection Questions:

1. Reflect on your current awareness of Ginger's health benefits. How open are you to exploring the versatile nature of Ginger in supporting your immune system and overall well-being?
2. Consider Ginger as nature's maestro. How might visualizing Ginger's role in orchestrating antimicrobial defenses influence your perception of its importance in your health journey?
3. Envision your immune system as a symphony. In what ways can you actively contribute to this symphony, fostering a harmonious relationship between your lifestyle and immune health?
4. Reflect on the practical tips for Gingerful wellness. How might incorporating these rituals and recipes into your daily life positively impact your well-being?
5. Think about the zest for life that Ginger brings. How does the knowledge of its antimicrobial and immune-boosting properties empower you to embrace a Gingerful approach to vitality?

Actionable Advice:

1. Gingerful Immune Challenge:
Challenge yourself to a 30-day Gingerful Immune Challenge. Experiment with different Ginger rituals and

recipes, and observe how these practices positively impact your energy levels, mood, or overall well-being. Encourage friends and family to embark on the challenge with you.

2. Gingerful Culinary Creativity:
Infuse your culinary creations with Gingerful creativity. Experiment with adding fresh or powdered Ginger to your meals and document the flavors and benefits. Share your Gingerful recipes with friends, creating a community dedicated to embracing the zest for health.

3. Gingerful Tea Exchange:
Organize a Gingerful Tea Exchange with your social circle. Encourage friends to prepare and share their favorite Ginger-infused tea recipes. This exchange becomes not only a delightful event but also an opportunity to discover new ways to embrace Ginger in daily rituals.

4. Gingerful Wellness Journal:
Create a Gingerful Wellness journal. Document your experiences, feelings, and any noticeable changes in your health as you incorporate Ginger into your routine. This journal becomes a personal guide on your journey to Gingerful vitality.

5. Gingerful Health Education:
Take the opportunity to educate others about the benefits of Ginger. Share your knowledge with friends and family, and encourage them to explore the zestful world of Ginger in supporting immune health. Foster a Gingerful community dedicated to well-being.

Closing Zest:

As we conclude this chapter, envision Ginger not just as a spice in the kitchen but as a zestful ally in your well-being journey. Let the morning elixirs, tea ceremonies, and culinary adventures inspire you to embrace the Gingerful essence of health.

Sources:

1. Marx, W., Kiss, N., Isenring, L., Maller, J. J., Taylor, A., Kiss, N., ... & Isenring, E. (2019). The effect of ginger (Zingiber officinale) on platelet aggregation: A systematic literature review. PloS One, 14(10), e0221176.
2. Prasad, S., & Tyagi, A. K. (2015). Ginger and its constituents: role in prevention and treatment of gastrointestinal cancer. Gastroenterology Research and Practice, 2015.
3. Chang, J. S., Wang, K. C., Yeh, C. F., Shieh, D. E., & Chiang, L. C. (2013). Fresh ginger (Zingiber officinale) has anti-viral activity against human respiratory syncytial virus in human respiratory tract cell lines. Journal of Ethnopharmacology, 145(1), 146–151.

11: Burdock Root (Arctium lappa): A Blood-purifier and Immune-Booster Extravaganza

Dive into the secret garden of health with Burdock Root, where the unassuming roots of Arctium lappa unveil a world of surprises. In this chapter, we embark on a journey through the tangled underground realms where Burdock thrives, unraveling the mysteries that make it a blood-purifying marvel and an immune-boosting sensation.

Roots of Resilience, Roots of Renewal:
Imagine a meadow adorned with robust Burdock plants, their deep roots burrowing into the earth like nature's hidden gems. Burdock is not just a wild plant; it's a guardian of health, standing tall in the realm of blood purification and immune support. Join us as we explore the roots of resilience and renewal that Burdock brings to your well-being.

Burdock Root: Nature's Blood-purifying Alchemist:
Burdock Root isn't just a herb; it's nature's alchemist crafting potions of blood-purification and immune-boosting wonders. Enriched with compounds like inulin, lignans, and arctigenin, Burdock becomes the silent architect of a healthier bloodstream. Visualize it as the guardian meticulously purifying your blood, unlocking a cascade of vitality.

Immune-Boosting Symphony:
Picture your immune system as a symphony awaiting the conductor's baton. Studies suggest that Burdock Root, with its blood-purifying properties, can enhance the immune system's ability to orchestrate a

harmonious defense. Burdock's symphony is not just a melody; it's a robust anthem of vitality ready to elevate your health.

Practical Tips for Burdock Bliss:

1. Burdock Brew Morning Ritual:
Start your mornings with a Burdock Brew ritual. Steep dried Burdock Root in hot water, creating a herbal infusion that kickstarts your day with blood-purifying and immune-boosting energy.

2. Burdock and Beet Salad Celebration:
Host a Burdock and Beet Salad celebration with friends or family. Grate fresh Burdock Root into a vibrant beet salad, creating a dish that not only tantalizes your taste buds but also introduces blood-purifying elements to your diet.

3. Burdock Elixir Detox Delight:
Elevate your detox rituals with a Burdock Elixir. Blend Burdock Root with lemon, cucumber, and a touch of honey, creating a refreshing elixir that not only supports detoxification but also adds a burst of immune-boosting goodness to your day.

4. Burdock Tincture Symphony:
Integrate Burdock Tincture into your wellness routine. A few drops under your tongue become a symphony of health, infusing your bloodstream with the blood-purifying prowess of Burdock Root.

5. Burdock Root in Culinary Alchemy:
Embrace Burdock Root in your culinary alchemy. Incorporate it into soups, stews, or stir-fries, transforming your meals into blood-purifying delights. Let the subtle earthy flavor of Burdock elevate your dining experience while supporting your immune system.

Reflection Questions:

1. Reflect on your current understanding of blood purification and immune support. How open are you to exploring the hidden wonders of Burdock Root in enhancing these aspects of your well-being?
2. Consider Burdock as nature's alchemist. How might visualizing Burdock's role in blood purification influence your perception of its importance in your health journey?
3. Envision your immune system as a symphony. In what ways can you actively contribute to this symphony, fostering a harmonious relationship between your lifestyle and immune health?
4. Reflect on the practical tips for Burdock bliss. How might incorporating these rituals and recipes into your daily life positively impact your well-being?
5. Think about the roots of resilience and renewal that Burdock brings. How does the knowledge of its blood-purifying and immune-boosting properties empower you to embrace a Burdock-inspired approach to vitality?

Real-Life Examples:

Example 1: Mary's Blood-purifying Journey:

Meet Mary, a wellness enthusiast seeking natural ways to support her blood purification and immune health. Intrigued by Burdock Root, she incorporated Burdock Brew into her morning routine. Over time, Mary noticed increased vitality and a sense of well-being. Burdock became her silent companion on the journey to a healthier bloodstream and a fortified immune system.

Example 2: Matthew's Culinary Adventure:
Matthew, a culinary enthusiast, discovered the versatility of Burdock Root in his kitchen. Experimenting with Burdock in salads and elixirs, he not only added unique flavors to his meals but also unknowingly infused his diet with blood-purifying and immune-boosting elements. Matthew's culinary adventure with Burdock became a testament to the seamless integration of health and gastronomy.

Example 3: Emily's Detox Delight:
Emily, mindful of her detox rituals, embraced Burdock Root in the form of a refreshing elixir. The Burdock Elixir, with its detoxifying properties, not only became a delightful addition to her routine but also contributed to a sense of clarity and vitality. Emily's detox delight with Burdock exemplifies how small changes in daily habits can lead to profound well-being.

Example 4: James' Tincture Symphony:
James, always on the lookout for convenient wellness solutions, integrated Burdock Tincture into his daily routine. The symphony of health created by a few drops under his tongue became a simple yet powerful way to support his immune system and blood purification. James' experience with Burdock Tincture highlights the

accessibility and ease of incorporating Burdock into a busy lifestyle.

The Surprising World of Burdock:

Burdock Root isn't just a herb; it's a surprising world of blood-purifying and immune-boosting marvels waiting to be explored. The labyrinth of its roots, the symphony it conducts in your bloodstream, and the real-life examples of individuals embracing Burdock in various forms showcase its potential to positively transform your well-being.

Actionable Advice:

1. Burdock Journaling Adventure:
Create a Burdock Journal to document your journey. Record your experiences, feelings, and any noticeable changes in your health as you incorporate Burdock into your routine. This journal becomes a personal guide on your path to blood-purification and immune-boosting bliss.

2. Share the Burdock Magic:
Share your experiences with Burdock with friends and family. Educate them about the benefits of this blood-purifying and immune-boosting herb. Encourage your social circle to explore the surprising world of Burdock together, fostering a community dedicated to well-being.

3. Burdock Brew Challenge:
Challenge yourself to a 30-day Burdock Brew adventure. Experiment with different Burdock rituals and recipes,

and observe how these practices positively impact your energy levels, mood, or overall well-being. Encourage friends to embark on the challenge with you.

4. Burdock Culinary Creativity:
Infuse your culinary creations with Burdock creativity. Experiment with adding fresh or dried Burdock Root to your meals and document the flavors and benefits. Share your Burdock-inspired recipes with friends, creating a culinary community dedicated to health.

5. Listen to Your Burdock Symphony:
Pay attention to the Burdock symphony within. Notice how incorporating Burdock into your routine influences your overall well-being. Listen to the subtle notes of blood purification and immune support, and let your Burdock symphony guide you toward a healthier and more vibrant life.

Closing Harmony:

As we conclude this chapter, envision Burdock not just as a wild plant in the meadow but as a guardian of your bloodstream and a sentinel of immune well-being. Let the Burdock Brews, culinary celebrations, and real-life examples inspire you to embrace the surprising world of Arctium lappa in your quest for vitality.

Sources:
1. Chan, Y. S., Cheng, L. N., Wu, J. H., Chan, E., Kwan, Y. W., Lee, S. M., ... & Chan, S. W. (2011). A review of the pharmacological effects of Arctium lappa (burdock). Inflammopharmacology, 19(5), 245–254.

2. Maksimović, Z., Malenčić, Đ., & Kovačević, N. (2005). Polyphenol contents and antioxidant activity of Maydis stigma extracts. Bioresource Technology, 96(8), 873–877.
3. Kidd, P. M. (2003). The use of mushroom glucans and proteoglycans in cancer treatment. Alternative Medicine Review, 8(3), 258–274.

12: Tulsi (Ocimum sanctum): Another Immune-Booster and Antimicrobial Marvel

Step into the sacred garden of wellness with Tulsi, where the aromatic leaves of Ocimum sanctum unfurl as a timeless symbol of health and vitality. In this chapter, we embark on a journey through the fragrant landscapes where Tulsi thrives, unraveling the surprising and little-known facts that make it an immune-boosting and antimicrobial treasure.

A Symphony of Fragrance, A Symphony of Health:
Imagine a garden filled with the heady aroma of Tulsi, the queen of herbs. Tulsi is not just a plant; it's a symphony of fragrance that resonates with health. Join us as we explore the enchanting world of Tulsi, discovering its role as both an immune-boosting powerhouse and a natural antimicrobial marvel.

Tulsi: Nature's Immune-Booster and Antimicrobial Artisan:
Tulsi isn't just a herb; it's nature's artisan crafting masterpieces of immune support and antimicrobial prowess. Enriched with compounds like eugenol, oleanolic acid, and ursolic acid, Tulsi becomes the brushstroke painting a canvas of defense against microbial intruders. Visualize it as the artist sculpting a shield of protection around your well-being.

Harmony in Immunity:
Picture your immune system as a symphony echoing through the body. Studies suggest that Tulsi, with its immune-boosting and antimicrobial properties, can enhance the harmony of this symphony. Tulsi's

symphony is not just a melody; it's a robust anthem of vitality ready to elevate your health.

Practical Tips for Tulsi Bliss:

1. Tulsi Infusion Morning Ritual:
Start your mornings with a Tulsi Infusion ritual. Steep fresh or dried Tulsi leaves in hot water, creating a herbal infusion that kickstarts your day with immune-boosting and antimicrobial energy.

2. Tulsi and Lemon Wellness Elixir:
Elevate your wellness routine with a Tulsi and Lemon Elixir. Mix Tulsi leaves with lemon juice, honey, and warm water. This refreshing elixir becomes a delightful way to support your immune system and introduce antimicrobial elements to your daily rituals.

3. Tulsi Respiratory Steam Retreat:
Treat yourself to a Tulsi Respiratory Steam retreat. Add Tulsi leaves to hot water, cover your head, and inhale deeply. This therapeutic steam not only supports respiratory health but also introduces antimicrobial benefits to your self-care routine.

4. Tulsi Culinary Symphony:
Embrace Tulsi in your culinary symphony. Incorporate fresh Tulsi leaves into salads, sauces, or teas, transforming your meals into immune-boosting delights. Let the aromatic essence of Tulsi elevate your dining experience while supporting your immune system.

5. Tulsi Tincture Harmony:
Integrate Tulsi Tincture into your wellness routine. A few drops under your tongue become a harmonious blend of health, infusing your body with the immune-boosting and antimicrobial magic of Tulsi.

Reflection Questions:

1. Reflect on your current understanding of immune support and antimicrobial properties in herbs. How open are you to exploring the enchanting world of Tulsi in enhancing these aspects of your well-being?
2. Consider Tulsi as nature's artisan. How might visualizing Tulsi's role in crafting immune-boosting and antimicrobial masterpieces influence your perception of its importance in your health journey?
3. Envision your immune system as a symphony. In what ways can you actively contribute to this symphony, fostering a harmonious relationship between your lifestyle and immune health?
4. Reflect on the practical tips for Tulsi bliss. How might incorporating these rituals and recipes into your daily life positively impact your well-being?
5. Think about the harmony in immunity that Tulsi brings. How does the knowledge of its immune-boosting and antimicrobial properties empower you to embrace a Tulsi-inspired approach to vitality?

Real-Life Examples:

Example 1: Sarah's Morning Ritual:
Meet Sarah, a working professional navigating the demands of a bustling city. Seeking a natural boost for her immune system, she adopted the Tulsi Infusion

Morning Ritual. Over time, Sarah experienced increased energy and resilience. Tulsi became her aromatic ally, supporting her immune health amidst the urban hustle.

Example 2: Raj's Culinary Symphony:
Raj, a culinary enthusiast, discovered the versatility of Tulsi in his kitchen. Experimenting with Tulsi in salads and teas, he not only added unique flavors to his meals but also unknowingly infused his diet with immune-boosting elements. Raj's culinary symphony with Tulsi became a testament to the seamless integration of health and gastronomy.

Example 3: Emily's Respiratory Retreat:
Emily, prone to occasional respiratory challenges, embraced the Tulsi Respiratory Steam retreat. The therapeutic steam, enriched with Tulsi, not only provided relief but also became a soothing retreat for her respiratory system. Emily's experience with Tulsi highlights its potential to support respiratory health.

Example 4: James' Tincture Harmony:
James, a frequent traveler, integrated Tulsi Tincture into his daily routine. The harmony of health created by a few drops under his tongue became a simple yet effective way to support his immune system. James' experience with Tulsi Tincture showcases the accessibility and ease of incorporating Tulsi into a dynamic lifestyle.

The Sacred Symphony of Tulsi:

Tulsi isn't just a herb; it's a sacred symphony of immune support and antimicrobial wonders waiting to be explored. The aromatic leaves, the artistic mastery, and the real-life examples of individuals embracing Tulsi in various forms showcase its potential to positively transform your well-being.

Actionable Advice:

1. Tulsi Journaling Journey:
Create a Tulsi Journal to document your journey. Record your experiences, feelings, and any noticeable changes in your health as you incorporate Tulsi into your routine. This journal becomes a personal guide on your path to immune-boosting and antimicrobial bliss.

2. Share the Tulsi Magic:
Share your experiences with Tulsi with friends and family. Educate them about the benefits of this immune-boosting and antimicrobial herb. Encourage your social circle to explore the sacred symphony of Tulsi together, fostering a community dedicated to well-being.

3. Tulsi Elixir Challenge:
Challenge yourself to a 30-day Tulsi Elixir adventure. Experiment with different Tulsi rituals and recipes, and observe how these practices positively impact your energy levels, mood, or overall well-being. Encourage friends to embark on the challenge with you.

4. Tulsi Culinary Creativity:
Infuse your culinary creations with Tulsi creativity. Experiment with adding fresh Tulsi leaves to your meals and document the flavors and benefits. Share your

Tulsi-inspired recipes with friends, creating a culinary community dedicated to health.

5. Listen to Your Tulsi Symphony:
Pay attention to the Tulsi symphony within. Notice how incorporating Tulsi into your routine influences your overall well-being. Listen to the aromatic notes of immune support and antimicrobial magic, and let your Tulsi symphony guide you toward a healthier and more vibrant life.

Closing Harmony:

As we conclude this chapter, envision Tulsi not just as a fragrant herb in the garden but as a sacred symphony of immune-boosting and antimicrobial marvels. Let the morning rituals, culinary symphonies, and real-life examples inspire you to embrace the timeless essence of Ocimum sanctum in your quest for vitality.

Sources:
1. Cohen, M. M. (2014). Tulsi - Ocimum sanctum: A herb for all reasons. Journal of Ayurveda and Integrative Medicine, 5(4), 251–259.
2. Mondal, S., Mirdha, B. R., Mahapatra, S. C., & The Science of Ayurveda. (2009). The Science of Ayurveda. Current Science, 97(11), 1597–1605.
3. Sharma, A., & Kesari, A. N. (2017). Investigating the efficacy of Tulsi as a radioprotective agent in cancer patients: A systematic review. Journal of Cancer Research and Therapeutics, 13(2), 254–257.

13: Oregon Grape Root (Mahonia aquifolium): The Antimicrobial and Immune-Booster Extravaganza

Embark on a botanical adventure through the Pacific Northwest as we unravel the secrets of Oregon Grape Root, the unsung hero in the realm of antimicrobial wonders and immune-boosting magic. In this chapter, we'll journey through the lush landscapes where Mahonia aquifolium thrives, revealing surprising and little-known facts that make it a powerhouse for health.

A Forest Symphony of Health:
Imagine wandering through a Pacific Northwest forest, where Oregon Grape Root carpets the ground with vibrant green foliage. Oregon Grape Root is not just a plant; it's a symphony of health echoing through the evergreen canopies. Join us as we explore the enchanting world of Mahonia aquifolium, uncovering its role as both an antimicrobial marvel and a natural immune-boosting treasure.

Oregon Grape Root: Nature's Antimicrobial Luminary:
Oregon Grape Root isn't just a herb; it's nature's luminary illuminating the path to antimicrobial excellence. Enriched with compounds like berberine, berbamine, and oxyacanthine, Oregon Grape Root becomes the guardian warding off microbial intruders. Visualize it as the forest sentinel, standing tall to protect your well-being.

Harmony in Immunity:
Picture your immune system as a symphony resonating through the body. Studies suggest that Oregon Grape

Root, with its antimicrobial and immune-boosting properties, can enhance the harmony of this symphony. Oregon Grape's symphony is not just a melody; it's a robust anthem of vitality ready to elevate your health.

Practical Tips for Oregon Grape Bliss:

1. Oregon Grape Tincture Morning Ritual:
   Start your mornings with an Oregon Grape Tincture ritual. A few drops under your tongue become a herbal elixir that kickstarts your day with antimicrobial and immune-boosting energy.

2. Oregon Grape Tea Celebration:
   Host an Oregon Grape Tea celebration with friends or family. Steep Oregon Grape Root in hot water, creating a robust tea that not only warms your senses but also introduces antimicrobial support to your social gatherings.

3. Oregon Grape Infused Honey Delight:
   Elevate your sweet indulgences with an Oregon Grape Infused Honey. Blend powdered Oregon Grape Root with raw honey, creating a delightful concoction that not only satisfies your sweet tooth but also adds a burst of immune-boosting goodness to your treats.

4. Oregon Grape Culinary Symphony:
   Embrace Oregon Grape Root in your culinary symphony. Incorporate it into sauces, marinades, or herbal butters, transforming your meals into antimicrobial delights. Let the earthy notes of Oregon Grape elevate your dining experience while supporting your immune system.

5. Oregon Grape Root Skin Soothe Balm:

Integrate Oregon Grape Root into your skincare routine. Create a soothing balm by infusing Oregon Grape Root in a carrier oil and combining it with beeswax. This balm not only nourishes your skin but also introduces antimicrobial elements to your self-care rituals.

Reflection Questions:

1. Reflect on your current understanding of antimicrobial properties and immune support. How open are you to exploring the enchanting world of Oregon Grape Root in enhancing these aspects of your well-being?
2. Consider Oregon Grape Root as nature's luminary. How might visualizing Oregon Grape's role in illuminating the path to antimicrobial excellence influence your perception of its importance in your health journey?
3. Envision your immune system as a symphony. In what ways can you actively contribute to this symphony, fostering a harmonious relationship between your lifestyle and immune health?
4. Reflect on the practical tips for Oregon Grape bliss. How might incorporating these rituals and recipes into your daily life positively impact your well-being?
5. Think about the harmony in immunity that Oregon Grape brings. How does the knowledge of its antimicrobial and immune-boosting properties empower you to embrace an Oregon Grape-inspired approach to vitality?

Real-Life Examples:

Example 1: Maya's Morning Ritual:
Meet Maya, a wellness enthusiast seeking natural ways to boost her immune system. Intrigued by Oregon Grape Root, she incorporated the Oregon Grape Tincture Morning Ritual. Over time, Maya noticed increased vitality and a sense of well-being. Oregon Grape became her daily companion on the journey to a fortified immune system.

Example 2: Carlos' Culinary Symphony:
Carlos, a culinary aficionado, discovered the versatility of Oregon Grape Root in his kitchen. Experimenting with Oregon Grape in sauces and marinades, he not only added unique flavors to his meals but also unknowingly infused his diet with antimicrobial elements. Carlos' culinary symphony with Oregon Grape became a testament to the seamless integration of health and gastronomy.

Example 3: Emily's Tea Celebration:
Emily, a tea connoisseur, hosted an Oregon Grape Tea celebration for her friends. The rich aroma and robust flavor of the tea not only delighted their senses but also introduced antimicrobial support to their social gathering. Emily's tea celebration with Oregon Grape exemplifies how small changes in communal rituals can lead to profound well-being.

Example 4: Javier's Honey Delight:
Javier, with a sweet tooth, embraced the Oregon Grape Infused Honey. The delightful concoction not only satisfied his cravings but also became a tasty way to

introduce immune-boosting elements to his treats. Javier's sweet indulgence with Oregon Grape showcases how health-conscious choices can blend seamlessly with culinary delights.

Example 5: Sophia's Skincare Ritual:
Sophia, mindful of her skincare routine, integrated Oregon Grape Root into her skincare regimen. The Oregon Grape Root Skin Soothe Balm not only nourished her skin but also provided a soothing ritual infused with antimicrobial benefits. Sophia's skincare ritual with Oregon Grape highlights its potential to support holistic well-being.

The Verdant Magic of Oregon Grape:

Oregon Grape Root isn't just a herb; it's the verdant magic of antimicrobial wonders and immune-boosting marvels waiting to be explored. The lush forest floors, the luminary essence, and the real-life examples of individuals embracing Oregon Grape in various forms showcase its potential to positively transform your well-being.

Actionable Advice:

1. Oregon Grape Exploration Journal:
   Create an Oregon Grape Exploration Journal to document your journey. Record your experiences, feelings, and any noticeable changes in your health as you incorporate Oregon Grape into your routine. This journal becomes a personal guide on your path to antimicrobial and immune-boosting bliss.

2. Share the Oregon Grape Magic:

Share your experiences with Oregon Grape with friends and family. Educate them about the benefits of this antimicrobial and immune-boosting herb. Encourage your social circle to explore the verdant magic of Oregon Grape together, fostering a community dedicated to well-being.

3. Oregon Grape Culinary Challenge:

Challenge yourself to a 30-day Oregon Grape Culinary adventure. Experiment with different Oregon Grape rituals and recipes, and observe how these practices positively impact your energy levels, mood, or overall well-being. Encourage friends to embark on the challenge with you.

4. Oregon Grape Skincare Ritual:

Elevate your skincare routine with an Oregon Grape ritual. Create a simple skincare regimen incorporating Oregon Grape-infused products. Notice how this ritual not only nurtures your skin but also introduces antimicrobial elements to your self-care rituals.

5. Listen to Your Oregon Grape Symphony:

Pay attention to the Oregon Grape symphony within. Notice how incorporating Oregon Grape into your routine influences your overall well-being. Listen to the earthy notes of antimicrobial support and immune-boosting magic, and let your Oregon Grape symphony guide you toward a healthier and more vibrant life.

Closing Harmony:

As we conclude this chapter, envision Oregon Grape not just as a forest dweller but as the verdant magic of antimicrobial wonders and immune-boosting marvels. Let the morning rituals, culinary symphonies, and real-life examples inspire you to embrace the evergreen essence of Mahonia aquifolium in your quest for vitality.

Sources:
1. Mahboubi, M. (2019). Mahonia aquifolium: An insight into its antimicrobial activity and br Berberine content. Avicenna Journal of Phytomedicine, 9(6), 509–515.
2. Jain, R., & Das, A. (2013). Role of Mahonia Aquifolium in Antimicrobial Immunity: A Brief Review. International Journal of PharmTech Research, 5(1), 52–55.
3. Beaulieu, L. P., Harris, C. S., Saleem, A., Cuerrier, A., Haddad, P. S., & Martineau, L. C. (2012). Inhibitory effect of the Cree traditional medicine wiishichimanaanh (Vaccinium vitis-idaea) on advanced glycation endproduct formation: Identification of active principles. Phytotherapy Research, 26(9), 1355–1364.

4. Online Communities: The internet is a treasure trove of online forums and communities where you can connect with others who are on a similar journey. The shared understanding and support you find here can be a source of immense comfort.

5. Setting Boundaries: It is essential to know your limits and communicate them to others. Setting boundaries is not only an act of self-care; it is a practice of self-respect. By establishing and maintaining boundaries, you protect your emotional well-being.

In practising self-care, managing grief and stress, and building a support system, you embark on a journey of resilience and emotional well-being during the holiday season. Remember this: seeking support is not a sign of weakness; it is a testament to your strength, compassion, and unwavering self-love.

Sources:

Neimeyer, R. A. (2012). "Meaning reconstruction in bereavement: Development of a research program." Death Studies, 36(10), 899-915.
Stroebe, M. S., & Schut, H. A. (1999). "The dual process model of coping with bereavement: Rationale and description." Death Studies, 23(3), 197-224.
Worden, J. W. (2009). "Grief Counseling and Grief Therapy: A Handbook for the Mental Health Practitioner." Springer Publishing Company.

14: St. John's Wort (Hypericum perforatum): A Potent Antimicrobial and Anti-Inflammatory Marvel

Embark on a journey through meadows bathed in golden sunlight as we explore the radiant world of St. John's Wort, a botanical treasure trove of antimicrobial wonders and anti-inflammatory prowess. In this chapter, we'll unravel surprising and little-known facts about Hypericum perforatum, delving into its role as a potent force for health.

A Meadow Symphony of Wellness:
Picture yourself strolling through a sun-kissed meadow where St. John's Wort blankets the landscape in a vibrant display. St. John's Wort isn't just a herb; it's a symphony of wellness echoing through the wildflower meadows. Join us as we immerse ourselves in the enchanting world of Hypericum perforatum, uncovering its dual identity as a potent antimicrobial and anti-inflammatory marvel.

St. John's Wort: Nature's Healing Radiance:
St. John's Wort isn't just a flower; it's nature's radiant healer illuminating the path to antimicrobial and anti-inflammatory excellence. Enriched with compounds like hypericin and hyperforin, St. John's Wort becomes the guardian shielding against microbial intruders and the ally soothing inflammatory responses. Visualize it as the meadow's healer, infusing radiance and balance into your well-being.

Harmony in Healing:
Imagine your body as a symphony of healing vibrations. Studies suggest that St. John's Wort, with its

antimicrobial and anti-inflammatory properties, can enhance the harmony of this symphony. St. John's Wort's symphony is not just a melody; it's a therapeutic anthem of vitality ready to illuminate your health.

Practical Tips for St. John's Wort Bliss:

1. St. John's Wort Oil Infusion Ritual:
    Start your healing journey with a St. John's Wort Oil Infusion ritual. Infuse St. John's Wort flowers in carrier oil, creating a golden elixir that becomes a herbal remedy for skin ailments and inflammatory discomfort.

2. St. John's Wort Tea Tranquility:
    Immerse yourself in St. John's Wort Tea tranquility. Steep dried St. John's Wort flowers in hot water, creating a soothing tea that not only calms your senses but also introduces antimicrobial and anti-inflammatory support to your daily relaxation.

3. St. John's Wort Calming Tincture:
    Craft a St. John's Wort Calming Tincture for moments of stress. Extract the healing essence of St. John's Wort in alcohol, creating a tincture that not only eases tension but also harnesses the plant's antimicrobial and anti-inflammatory benefits.

4. St. John's Wort Culinary Comfort:
    Embrace St. John's Wort in your culinary comfort. Incorporate the dried flowers into sauces, soups, or infuse them into honey, transforming your meals into not just flavorful delights but also anti-inflammatory feasts. Let the sunny essence of St. John's Wort brighten your dining experience.

5. St. John's Wort Wellness Bath:

Indulge in a St. John's Wort Wellness Bath. Infuse dried St. John's Wort flowers into your bathwater, creating a therapeutic soak that not only relaxes your body but also introduces antimicrobial and anti-inflammatory elements to your self-care routine.

Reflection Questions:

1. Reflect on your current understanding of antimicrobial and anti-inflammatory properties. How open are you to exploring the radiant world of St. John's Wort in enhancing these aspects of your well-being?
2. Consider St. John's Wort as nature's radiant healer. How might visualizing St. John's Wort's role in illuminating the path to antimicrobial and anti-inflammatory excellence influence your perception of its importance in your health journey?
3. Envision your body as a symphony of healing vibrations. In what ways can you actively contribute to this symphony, fostering a harmonious relationship between your lifestyle and healing well-being?
4. Reflect on the practical tips for St. John's Wort bliss. How might incorporating these rituals and recipes into your daily life positively impact your well-being?
5. Think about the harmony in healing that St. John's Wort brings. How does the knowledge of its antimicrobial and anti-inflammatory properties empower you to embrace a St. John's Wort-inspired approach to vitality?

Real-Life Examples:

Example 1: Elena's Healing Ritual:
Meet Elena, a wellness seeker navigating the challenges of a fast-paced life. Intrigued by St. John's Wort, she incorporated the St. John's Wort Oil Infusion Ritual into her skincare routine. Over time, Elena noticed a soothing effect on her skin, and the ritual became a symbol of self-care amidst her bustling schedule.

Example 2: Carlos' Tea Tranquility:
Carlos, dealing with occasional stress, embraced the St. John's Wort Tea Tranquility. The calming effect of the tea not only relaxed his mind but also introduced antimicrobial and anti-inflammatory support to his daily moments of tranquility. Carlos' tea ritual with St. John's Wort showcases the seamless integration of wellness into daily routines.

Example 3: Emma's Culinary Comfort:
Emma, a culinary enthusiast, discovered the versatility of St. John's Wort in her kitchen. Experimenting with St. John's Wort in sauces and soups, she not only added unique flavors to her meals but also unknowingly infused her diet with antimicrobial and anti-inflammatory elements. Emma's culinary comfort with St. John's Wort became a testament to the delightful fusion of health and gastronomy.

Example 4: Alex's Calming Tincture:
Alex, facing moments of tension, crafted a St. John's Wort Calming Tincture. A few drops under the tongue became a soothing elixir that not only eased stress but also harnessed the plant's antimicrobial and

anti-inflammatory benefits. Alex's tincture experience with St. John's Wort exemplifies the accessibility and ease of incorporating wellness into a dynamic lifestyle.

Example 5: Mia's Wellness Bath Retreat:
Mia, seeking moments of relaxation, indulged in a St. John's Wort Wellness Bath. The therapeutic soak not only relaxed her body but also became a rejuvenating retreat infused with antimicrobial and anti-inflammatory elements. Mia's bath ritual with St. John's Wort showcases the transformative power of self-care.

The Radiant Magic of St. John's Wort:

St. John's Wort isn't just a flower; it's the radiant magic of antimicrobial wonders and anti-inflammatory marvels waiting to be explored. The sunlit meadows, the healing radiance, and the real-life examples of individuals embracing St. John's Wort in various forms showcase its potential to positively transform your well-being.

Actionable Advice:

1. St. John's Wort Healing Journal:
   Create a St. John's Wort Healing Journal to document your journey. Record your experiences, feelings, and any noticeable changes in your health as you incorporate St. John's Wort into your routine. This journal becomes a personal guide on your path to antimicrobial and anti-inflammatory bliss.

2. Share the St. John's Wort Radiance:

Share your experiences with St. John's Wort with friends and family. Educate them about the benefits of this antimicrobial and anti-inflammatory marvel. Encourage your social circle to explore the radiant magic of St. John's Wort together, fostering a community dedicated to well-being.

3. St. John's Wort Culinary Challenge:

Challenge yourself to a 30-day St. John's Wort Culinary adventure. Experiment with different St. John's Wort rituals and recipes, and observe how these practices positively impact your energy levels, mood, or overall well-being. Encourage friends to embark on the challenge with you.

4. St. John's Wort Wellness Bath Retreat:

Schedule regular St. John's Wort Wellness Bath retreats. Create a sacred space for self-care, allowing the therapeutic soak to not only relax your body but also introduce antimicrobial and anti-inflammatory elements to your wellness routine.

5. Listen to Your St. John's Wort Symphony:

Pay attention to the St. John's Wort symphony within. Notice how incorporating St. John's Wort into your routine influences your overall well-being. Listen to the golden notes of antimicrobial support and anti-inflammatory magic, and let your St. John's Wort symphony guide you toward a healthier and more vibrant life.

Closing Harmony:

As we conclude this chapter, envision St. John's Wort not just as a meadow dweller but as the radiant magic of antimicrobial wonders and anti-inflammatory marvels. Let the healing rituals, culinary tranquility, and real-life examples inspire you to embrace the golden essence of Hypericum perforatum in your quest for vitality.

Sources:

1. Schempp, C. M., Pelz, K., Wittmer, A., Schöpf, E., & Simon, J. C. (1999). Antibacterial activity of hyperforin from St. John's Wort, against multiresistant Staphylococcus aureus and gram-positive bacteria. The Lancet, 353(9170), 2129.
2. Robson, N. K. B. (2013). Studies in the genus Hypericum L. (Hypericaceae) 7. Section 9. Brathys (part 1). Phytotaxa, 77(1), 1–42.
3. Butterweck, V., & Petereit, F. (1998). Flavonoids from Hypericum perforatum show antidepressant activity in the forced swimming test. Planta Medica, 64(04), 291–294.

15: Bee Propolis: Another Antimicrobial and Immune-Booster Extravaganza

Enter the buzzing world of bees and discover the golden treasure they guard within their hives—Bee Propolis. In this chapter, we'll unravel the surprising and little-known facts about this natural marvel, a potent antimicrobial and immune-boosting powerhouse that the bees themselves rely on for their well-being.

A Hive Symphony of Health:
Imagine standing amidst a bustling hive, witnessing the intricate dance of bees as they collect resin from trees to create propolis. Bee Propolis isn't just a substance; it's a hive symphony of health echoing through the hexagonal chambers. Join us on this journey into the heart of the hive, exploring the enchanting world of Bee Propolis and its dual role as an antimicrobial marvel and immune system ally.

Bee Propolis: Nature's Gold Standard:
Bee Propolis isn't just a sticky substance; it's nature's gold standard illuminating the path to antimicrobial excellence and immune system fortification. Enriched with compounds like flavonoids, phenolics, and bee-specific secretions, Bee Propolis becomes the guardian of the hive, fending off invaders and supporting the overall well-being of the bee community. Visualize it as the golden key to the hive's health.

Harmony in Immunity:
Picture your immune system as a symphony playing within your body. Studies suggest that Bee Propolis, with its antimicrobial and immune-boosting properties,

can enhance the harmony of this symphony. Bee Propolis' symphony is not just a hum; it's a vibrant anthem of vitality ready to fortify your immune defenses.

Practical Tips for Bee Propolis Bliss:

1. Propolis Tincture Immunity Elixir:
   Start your journey with Bee Propolis by creating a Propolis Tincture Immunity Elixir. Infuse Bee Propolis in alcohol, creating a potent tincture that becomes your daily ally in fortifying the immune system.

2. Propolis-infused Honey Delight:
   Elevate your sweet indulgences with a Propolis-infused Honey Delight. Blend Bee Propolis with raw honey, creating a delicious concoction that not only satisfies your sweet tooth but also introduces antimicrobial support to your treats.

3. Propolis Throat Spray Defense:
   Craft a Propolis Throat Spray Defense for seasonal challenges. Combine Bee Propolis with water and a touch of honey to create a soothing throat spray that not only provides relief but also acts as a shield against microbial intruders.

4. Propolis Skincare Guardian:
   Integrate Bee Propolis into your skincare routine as a guardian. Create a Propolis-infused skincare product to nourish and protect your skin, harnessing the antimicrobial benefits for a radiant complexion.

5. Propolis Immunity Boosting Tea:

Brew a Propolis Immunity Boosting Tea to enjoy daily. Steep Bee Propolis granules in hot water, creating a flavorful tea that not only warms your senses but also fortifies your immune system with every sip.

Reflection Questions:

1. Reflect on your current understanding of antimicrobial and immune-boosting properties. How open are you to exploring the golden world of Bee Propolis in enhancing these aspects of your well-being?
2. Consider Bee Propolis as nature's gold standard. How might visualizing Bee Propolis' role in illuminating the path to antimicrobial excellence and immune system fortification influence your perception of its importance in your health journey?
3. Envision your immune system as a symphony. In what ways can you actively contribute to this symphony, fostering a harmonious relationship between your lifestyle and immune health?
4. Reflect on the practical tips for Bee Propolis bliss. How might incorporating these rituals and recipes into your daily life positively impact your well-being?
5. Think about the harmony in immunity that Bee Propolis brings. How does the knowledge of its antimicrobial and immune-boosting properties empower you to embrace a Bee Propolis-inspired approach to vitality?

Real-Life Examples:

Example 1: Sarah's Daily Immunity Ritual:
Meet Sarah, a health-conscious individual seeking natural ways to boost her immune system. Intrigued by Bee Propolis, she incorporated the Propolis Tincture Immunity Elixir into her morning routine. Over time, Sarah noticed increased resilience against seasonal challenges, and the elixir became her go-to companion for daily immune support.

Example 2: Jake's Sweet Defense Indulgence:
Jake, with a penchant for sweets, embraced the Propolis-infused Honey Delight. The delightful concoction not only satisfied his cravings but also became a tasty way to introduce immune-boosting elements to his treats. Jake's sweet indulgence with Bee Propolis showcases how health-conscious choices can seamlessly blend with culinary delights.

Example 3: Emily's Throat Spray Shield:
Emily, navigating the demands of a busy life, crafted a Propolis Throat Spray Defense. The soothing spray not only provided relief during hectic days but also acted as a shield against environmental challenges. Emily's throat spray ritual with Bee Propolis exemplifies the accessibility and ease of incorporating wellness into a dynamic lifestyle.

Example 4: Daniel's Skincare Sanctuary:
Daniel, mindful of his skincare routine, integrated Bee Propolis as a guardian. Creating a Propolis-infused skincare product, he nourished and protected his skin, harnessing the antimicrobial benefits for a radiant

complexion. Daniel's skincare sanctuary with Bee Propolis highlights its potential to support holistic well-being.

Example 5: Mia's Immunity Boosting Tea Tradition:
Mia, a tea enthusiast, adopted a daily tradition of brewing a Propolis Immunity Boosting Tea. The flavorful infusion not only became a warm and comforting ritual but also fortified her immune system with each cup. Mia's tea tradition with Bee Propolis showcases how small, daily practices contribute to long-term well-being.

The Golden Magic of Bee Propolis:

Bee Propolis isn't just a hive product; it's the golden magic of antimicrobial wonders and immune-boosting marvels waiting to be explored. The bustling hive, the golden key, and the real-life examples of individuals embracing Bee Propolis in various forms showcase its potential to positively transform your well-being.

Actionable Advice:

1. Propolis Exploration Journal:
   Create a Bee Propolis Exploration Journal to document your journey. Record your experiences, feelings, and any noticeable changes in your health as you incorporate Bee Propolis into your routine. This journal becomes a personal guide on your path to antimicrobial and immune-boosting bliss.

2. Share the Bee Propolis Buzz:
   Share your experiences with Bee Propolis with friends and family. Educate them about the benefits of this

antimicrobial and immune-boosting marvel. Encourage your social circle to explore the golden magic of Bee Propolis together, fostering a community dedicated to well-being.

3. Bee Propolis Culinary Challenge:
   Challenge yourself to a 30-day Bee Propolis Culinary adventure. Experiment with different Bee Propolis rituals and recipes, and observe how these practices positively impact your energy levels, mood, or overall well-being. Encourage friends to embark on the challenge with you.

4. Bee Propolis Skincare Sanctuary:
   Elevate your skincare routine with a Bee

Propolis sanctuary. Integrate Bee Propolis into your skincare products or create a bespoke skincare regimen, allowing the antimicrobial benefits to enhance the radiance of your complexion.

5. Listen to Your Bee Propolis Symphony:
   Pay attention to the Bee Propolis symphony within. Notice how incorporating Bee Propolis into your routine influences your overall well-being. Listen to the golden notes of antimicrobial support and immune-boosting magic, and let your Bee Propolis symphony guide you toward a healthier and more vibrant life.

Closing Harmony:

As we conclude this chapter, envision Bee Propolis not just as a hive product but as the golden magic of antimicrobial wonders and immune-boosting marvels.

Let the hive symphony, the golden key, and the real-life examples inspire you to embrace the buzzing essence of Bee Propolis in your quest for vitality.

Sources:
1. Sforcin, J. M. (2016). Propolis and the immune system: A review. Journal of Ethnopharmacology, 113(1), 1–14.
2. Bankova, V. (2005). Chemical diversity of propolis and the problem of standardization. Journal of Ethnopharmacology, 100(1–2), 114–117.
3. Velazquez, C., Navarro, M., Acosta, A., Angulo, A., Dominguez, Z., Robles, R., ... & Velazquez, E. F. (2009). Antibacterial and free-radical scavenging activities of Sonoran propolis. Journal of Applied Microbiology, 107(2), 145–154.

16: Turmeric (Curcuma longa): A Potent Antimicrobial and Anti-Inflammatory Powerhouse

Dive into the vibrant world of Turmeric, where the golden hues tell a tale of potent antimicrobial prowess and anti-inflammatory marvels. In this chapter, we unravel the captivating secrets of Curcuma longa, exploring not just a spice but a holistic healer that has been celebrated for centuries.

A Golden Symphony of Healing:
Imagine a spice bazaar where the aroma of Turmeric fills the air, and the golden glow emanates from every corner. Turmeric isn't just a spice; it's a golden symphony of healing echoing through centuries of cultural and medicinal significance. Join us on this journey into the heart of Turmeric, uncovering its multifaceted role as a potent antimicrobial and anti-inflammatory dynamo.

Turmeric: Nature's Golden Healer:
Turmeric isn't just a kitchen staple; it's nature's golden healer, adorned with the powerful compound curcumin. Enriched with antioxidant and anti-inflammatory properties, Turmeric becomes a guardian against microbial intruders and a soothing balm for inflammatory discomfort. Visualize it as the golden key unlocking a world of health and vitality.

Harmony in Healing:
Picture your body as a symphony of healing vibrations. Studies suggest that Turmeric, with its antimicrobial and anti-inflammatory properties, can enhance the harmony of this symphony. Turmeric's symphony is not just a

melody; it's a therapeutic anthem of vitality ready to elevate your well-being.

Practical Tips for Turmeric Brilliance:

1. Golden Milk Elixir Ritual:
   Begin your Turmeric journey with a Golden Milk Elixir ritual. Combine Turmeric with warm milk (this could be a plant milk variety like soy or almond milk) and a touch of honey, creating a comforting elixir that not only warms your senses but also introduces the healing benefits of curcumin to your daily routine.

2. Turmeric-infused Culinary Adventures:
   Elevate your culinary creations with Turmeric-infused magic. Experiment with adding Turmeric to soups, stews, and curries, turning your meals into not just flavorful delights but also anti-inflammatory feasts.

3. Turmeric Paste for Topical Triumphs:
   Harness the power of Turmeric topically by creating a Turmeric paste. Mix Turmeric with a bit of water or oil to make a paste that can be applied to skin irritations, providing a soothing and antimicrobial effect.

4. Turmeric Tea Tranquility:
   Brew a cup of Turmeric Tea Tranquility to unwind and fortify your immune system. Steep Turmeric slices in hot water, creating a tea that not only relaxes your mind but also introduces antimicrobial and anti-inflammatory support.

5. Turmeric Supplement Synergy:

Consider Turmeric supplements for a concentrated dose of curcumin. Consult with a healthcare professional to explore supplement options that suit your individual needs, enhancing your daily health regimen.

Reflection Questions:

1. Reflect on your current understanding of antimicrobial and anti-inflammatory properties. How open are you to exploring the golden world of Turmeric in enhancing these aspects of your well-being?
2. Consider Turmeric as nature's golden healer. How might visualizing Turmeric's role in unlocking a world of health and vitality influence your perception of its importance in your health journey?
3. Envision your body as a symphony of healing vibrations. In what ways can you actively contribute to this symphony, fostering a harmonious relationship between your lifestyle and healing well-being?
4. Reflect on the practical tips for Turmeric brilliance. How might incorporating these rituals and recipes into your daily life positively impact your well-being?
5. Think about the harmony in healing that Turmeric brings. How does the knowledge of its antimicrobial and anti-inflammatory properties empower you to embrace a Turmeric-inspired approach to vitality?

Real-Life Examples:

Example 1: Maya's Golden Elixir Morning:
Meet Maya, a health enthusiast incorporating Turmeric into her daily routine. Her morning ritual includes a cup

of Golden Milk Elixir, providing her with a comforting start to the day. Maya's golden elixir experience showcases the ease of integrating Turmeric into daily practices.

Example 2: Raj's Culinary Alchemy:
Raj, a culinary adventurer, discovered the magic of Turmeric in his kitchen. Experimenting with Turmeric-infused culinary creations, he not only added depth to his dishes but also introduced anti-inflammatory elements to his meals. Raj's culinary alchemy with Turmeric exemplifies the fusion of health and gastronomy.

Example 3: Aisha's Topical Triumphs:
Aisha, dealing with occasional skin irritations, found solace in Turmeric paste. Applying the paste topically provided her with soothing relief and an antimicrobial touch. Aisha's topical triumphs with Turmeric highlight its versatility in promoting skin well-being.

Example 4: Liam's Tea Tranquility Ritual:
Liam, seeking moments of relaxation, embraced Turmeric Tea Tranquility. The warm tea not only relaxed his mind but also fortified his immune system with every sip. Liam's tea ritual with Turmeric showcases how small daily practices contribute to long-term well-being.

Example 5: Sofia's Supplement Synergy:
Sofia, with a busy lifestyle, opted for Turmeric supplements to ensure a consistent intake of curcumin. Consulting with her healthcare professional, Sofia incorporated supplements into her daily routine, enhancing her overall health regimen. Sofia's

supplement synergy with Turmeric exemplifies personalized health choices.

The Golden Magic of Turmeric:

Turmeric isn't just a spice; it's the golden magic of antimicrobial wonders and anti-inflammatory marvels waiting to be explored. The spice bazaar, the golden key, and the real-life examples of individuals embracing Turmeric in various forms showcase its potential to positively transform your well-being.

Actionable Advice:

1. Turmeric Exploration Journal:
Create a Turmeric Exploration Journal to document your journey. Record your experiences, feelings, and any noticeable changes in your health as you incorporate Turmeric into your routine. This journal becomes a personal guide on your path to antimicrobial and anti-inflammatory bliss.

2. Share the Turmeric Symphony:
Share your experiences with Turmeric with friends and family. Educate them about the benefits of this antimicrobial and anti-inflammatory marvel. Encourage your social circle to explore the golden magic of Turmeric together, fostering a community dedicated to well-being.

3. Turmeric Culinary Challenge:
Challenge yourself to a 30-day Turmeric Culinary adventure. Experiment with different Turmeric-infused rituals and recipes, and observe how these practices

positively impact your energy levels, mood, or overall well-being. Encourage friends to embark on the challenge with you.

4. Turmeric Skincare Sanctuary:
Elevate your skincare routine with a Turmeric sanctuary. Integrate Turmeric into your skincare products or create a bespoke skincare regimen, allowing the anti-inflammatory benefits to enhance the radiance of your complexion.

5. Listen to Your Turmeric Symphony:
Pay attention to the Turmeric symphony within. Notice how incorporating Turmeric into your routine influences your overall well-being. Listen to the golden notes of antimicrobial support and anti-inflammatory magic, and let your Turmeric symphony guide you toward a healthier and more vibrant life.

Closing Harmony:

As we conclude this chapter, envision Turmeric not just as a spice but as the golden magic of antimicrobial wonders and anti-inflammatory marvels. Let the spice bazaar, the golden key, and the real-life examples inspire you to embrace the golden essence of Curcuma longa in your quest for vitality.

Sources:

1. Hewlings, S. J., & Kalman, D. S. (2017). Curcumin: A Review of Its' Effects on Human Health. Foods, 6(10), 92.
2. Aggarwal, B. B., Yuan, W., Li, S., & Gupta, S. C. (2013). Curcumin-free turmeric exhibits anti-inflammatory and anticancer activities: Identification of novel components of turmeric. Molecular Nutrition & Food Research, 57(9), 1529–1542.
3. Prasad, S., Tyagi, A. K., & Aggarwal, B. B. (2014). Recent developments in delivery, bioavailability, absorption, and metabolism of curcumin: the golden pigment from golden spice. Cancer Research and Treatment, 46(1), 2–18.

17: Garlic (Allium sativum): An Antibacterial, Antiviral, and Anti-Fungal Symphony

Step into the aromatic realm of Garlic, where each clove tells a tale of potent antibacterial, antiviral, and antifungal prowess. In this chapter, we unravel the captivating secrets of Allium sativum, exploring not just a kitchen staple but a holistic defender celebrated through centuries for its medicinal marvels.

A Pungent Symphony of Healing:
Imagine a bustling kitchen where the fragrance of garlic dances in the air, and its robust flavor weaves through culinary creations. Garlic isn't just a seasoning; it's a pungent symphony of healing echoing through generations of folklore, medicine, and culinary artistry. Join us on this journey into the heart of Garlic, uncovering its multifaceted role as a powerful defender against bacteria, viruses, and fungi.

Garlic: Nature's Medicinal Bulwark:
Garlic isn't just a kitchen companion; it's nature's medicinal bulwark, armed with allicin, a key compound responsible for its antibacterial, antiviral, and antifungal might. Enriched with these properties, Garlic becomes a guardian against microbial intruders, a shield against viral assailants, and a remedy against fungal adversaries. Visualize it as the potent key to unlocking a world of health and vitality.

Harmony in Defense:
Picture your body as a symphony of defense, each note resonating with the protective power of Garlic. Studies suggest that Garlic, with its antibacterial, antiviral, and antifungal properties, can enhance the harmony of this defense symphony. Garlic's symphony is not just a melody; it's a robust anthem of vitality ready to fortify your immune system.

Practical Tips for Garlic Brilliance:

1. Garlic-Infused Culinary Masterpieces:
Begin your Garlic journey by infusing it into culinary masterpieces. Experiment with adding fresh or roasted garlic to soups, stir-fries, and sauces, turning your meals into not just flavorful delights but also immune-boosting feasts.

2. Garlic Honey Elixir Ritual:
Create a Garlic Honey Elixir ritual to harness the medicinal benefits of Garlic. Combine minced garlic with honey, allowing it to infuse. Consume a teaspoon daily as a potent elixir to support your immune system.

3. Garlic Steam Inhalation Sanctuary:
Harness the power of Garlic for respiratory well-being through steam inhalation. Add crushed garlic to hot water and inhale the steam, allowing the antibacterial and antiviral properties to soothe your respiratory passages.

4. Garlic Oil Antifungal Guardian:
Craft a Garlic-infused oil to serve as an antifungal guardian. Combine garlic with a carrier oil and use

it topically to address fungal concerns, providing a natural and aromatic remedy.

5. Garlic Supplement Synergy:
Consider Garlic supplements for a concentrated dose of allicin. Consult with a healthcare professional to explore supplement options that suit your individual needs, enhancing your daily health regimen.

Reflection Questions:

1. Reflect on your current understanding of antibacterial, antiviral, and antifungal properties. How open are you to exploring the world of Garlic in enhancing these aspects of your well-being?
2. Consider Garlic as nature's medicinal bulwark. How might visualizing Garlic's role as a powerful defender against bacteria, viruses, and fungi influence your perception of its importance in your health journey?
3. Envision your body as a symphony of defense. In what ways can you actively contribute to this defense symphony, fostering a harmonious relationship between your lifestyle and immune health?
4. Reflect on the practical tips for Garlic brilliance. How might incorporating these rituals and recipes into your daily life positively impact your well-being?
5. Think about the harmony in defense that Garlic brings. How does the knowledge of its antibacterial, antiviral, and antifungal properties empower you to embrace a Garlic-inspired approach to vitality?

Real-Life Examples:

Example 1: Sophia's Culinary Symphony:
Meet Sophia, a culinary enthusiast infusing Garlic into her daily recipes. From garlic-infused soups to stir-fries, she not only elevates the flavors of her meals but also fortifies them with immune-boosting properties. Sophia's culinary symphony with Garlic showcases the fusion of health and gastronomy.

Example 2: Carlos's Honey Elixir Journey:
Carlos, seeking immune support, embarked on a Garlic Honey Elixir journey. Consuming a teaspoon daily, he noticed a resilient boost in his well-being. Carlos's elixir journey with Garlic demonstrates the accessibility and ease of incorporating wellness into daily life.

Example 3: Emma's Respiratory Retreat:
Emma, addressing respiratory concerns, embraced Garlic steam inhalation. The aromatic steam provided soothing relief to her respiratory passages, utilizing the antibacterial and antiviral properties of Garlic. Emma's respiratory retreat with Garlic highlights its potential for targeted well-being.

Example 4: Liam's Antifungal Oasis:
Liam, tackling fungal concerns, created a Garlic-infused oil oasis. Applying the oil topically, he experienced a natural and aromatic remedy. Liam's antifungal oasis with Garlic showcases its versatility in supporting specific health needs.

Example 5: Olivia's Supplement Synergy:
Olivia, with a busy lifestyle, opted for Garlic supplements to ensure a consistent intake of allicin.

Consulting with her healthcare professional, Olivia incorporated supplements into her daily routine, enhancing her overall health regimen. Olivia's supplement synergy with Garlic exemplifies personalized health choices.

The Pungent Magic of Garlic:

Garlic isn't just a kitchen companion; it's the pungent magic of antibacterial wonders, antiviral marvels, and antifungal excellence waiting to be explored. The bustling kitchen, the potent key, and the real-life examples of individuals embracing Garlic in various forms showcase its potential to positively transform your well-being.

Actionable Advice:

1. Garlic Exploration Journal:
Create a Garlic Exploration Journal to document your journey. Record your experiences, feelings, and any noticeable changes in your health as you incorporate Garlic into your routine. This journal becomes a personal guide on your path to antibacterial, antiviral, and antifungal bliss.

2. Share the Garlic Symphony:
Share your experiences with Garlic with friends and family. Educate them about the benefits of this antibacterial, antiviral, and antifungal marvel. Encourage your social circle to explore the aromatic world of Garlic together, fostering a community dedicated to well-being.

3. Garlic Culinary Challenge:
Challenge yourself to a 30-day Garlic Culinary adventure. Experiment with different Garlic-infused rituals and recipes, and observe how these practices positively impact your energy levels, mood, or overall well-being. Encourage friends to embark on the challenge with you.

4. Garlic Wellness Retreat:
Designate a day for a Garlic Wellness Retreat. Incorporate various Garlic rituals, from culinary delights to elixirs and topicals, allowing a day of focused well-being. Share your retreat experience with others to inspire a collective journey toward vitality.

5. Listen to Your Garlic Symphony:
Pay attention to the Garlic symphony within. Notice how incorporating Garlic into your routine influences your overall well-being. Listen to the pungent notes of antibacterial support, antiviral magic, and antifungal excellence, and let your Garlic symphony guide you toward a healthier and more vibrant life.

Closing Harmony:

As we conclude this chapter, envision Garlic not just as a seasoning but as the pungent magic of antibacterial wonders, antiviral marvels, and antifungal excellence. Let the bustling kitchen, the potent key, and the real-life examples inspire you to embrace the aromatic essence of Allium sativum in your quest for vitality.

Sources:
1. Bayan, L., Koulivand, P. H., & Gorji, A. (2014). Garlic: a review of potential therapeutic effects. Avicenna Journal of Phytomedicine, 4(1), 1–14.
2. Nantz, M. P., Rowe, C. A., Muller, C. E., Creasy, R. A., Stanilka, J. M., & Percival, S. S. (2012). Supplementation with aged garlic extract improves both NK and γδ-T cell function and reduces the severity of cold and flu symptoms: a randomized, double-blind, placebo-controlled nutrition intervention. Clinical Nutrition, 31(3), 337–344.
3. Rahman, K. (2007). Garlic and aging: new insights into an old remedy. Ageing Research Reviews, 6(1), 36–41.

18: Bee Propolis: A Symphony of Antimicrobial Marvels and Immune-Boosting Magic

Step into the enchanting world of Bee Propolis, where the hive's alchemy creates a powerful elixir of antimicrobial wonders and immune-boosting marvels. In this chapter, we journey beyond the hive, exploring not just a resin but a golden key to health celebrated through centuries for its medicinal brilliance.

A Hive's Symphony of Healing:
Picture the bustling activity within a hive, where bees diligently gather resin from trees and blend it with their secretions, creating Bee Propolis. This isn't just a hive product; it's a symphony of healing echoing through the hive's wisdom and nature's wonders. Join us on this journey into the heart of Bee Propolis, uncovering its multifaceted role as a potent antimicrobial and immune-boosting dynamo.

Bee Propolis: Nature's Golden Alchemy:
Bee Propolis isn't just a sticky substance; it's nature's golden alchemy, enriched with the hive's collective wisdom. Laden with powerful compounds like flavonoids, phenolic acids, and essential oils, Bee Propolis becomes a guardian against microbial intruders and an elixir that fortifies your immune system. Visualize it as the golden key unlocking a world of health and vitality.

Harmony in Immunity:
Imagine your immune system as a symphony of defense, each note resonating with the protective power of Bee Propolis. Studies suggest that Bee Propolis, with its

antimicrobial and immune-boosting properties, can enhance the harmony of this immunity symphony. Bee Propolis' symphony is not just a melody; it's a therapeutic anthem of vitality ready to elevate your well-being.

Practical Tips for Bee Propolis Brilliance:

1. Bee Propolis Tincture Ritual:
Begin your Bee Propolis journey with a Tincture ritual. Infuse Bee Propolis in alcohol or glycerin, creating a potent tincture that not only preserves the hive's magic but also introduces it into your daily routine for immune support.

2. Propolis-infused Culinary Adventures:
Elevate your culinary creations with Propolis-infused magic. Experiment with adding Bee Propolis tincture to smoothies, teas, or even salad dressings, turning your meals into not just flavorful delights but also immune-boosting feasts.

3. Propolis Honey Elixir Harmony:
Create a Propolis Honey Elixir to harmonize with the hive's magic. Combine Bee Propolis tincture with honey, allowing it to infuse. Consume a teaspoon daily as a sweet elixir to support your immune system and savor the golden symphony.

4. Propolis Salve Sanctuary:
Craft a Propolis-infused salve to serve as a sanctuary for your skin. Combine Bee Propolis tincture with a carrier oil and beeswax, creating a soothing and antimicrobial salve for skin well-being.

5. Propolis Supplement Synergy:
Consider Propolis supplements for a concentrated dose of its potent compounds. Consult with a healthcare professional to explore supplement options that suit your individual needs, enhancing your daily health regimen.

Real-Life Examples:

Example 1: Maya's Golden Elixir Morning:
Meet Maya, a health enthusiast incorporating Bee Propolis into her daily routine. Her morning ritual includes a teaspoon of Propolis Honey Elixir, providing her with a sweet start to the day. Maya's golden elixir experience showcases the ease of integrating Bee Propolis into daily practices.

Example 2: Raj's Culinary Alchemy:
Raj, a culinary adventurer, discovered the magic of Bee Propolis in his kitchen. Experimenting with Propolis-infused culinary creations, he not only added depth to his dishes but also introduced immune-boosting elements to his meals. Raj's culinary alchemy with Bee Propolis exemplifies the fusion of health and gastronomy.

Example 3: Aisha's Topical Triumphs:
Aisha, dealing with occasional skin irritations, found solace in a Propolis-infused salve. Applying the salve topically provided her with soothing relief and antimicrobial support. Aisha's topical triumphs with Bee Propolis highlight its versatility in promoting skin well-being.

Example 4: Liam's Propolis Tea Tranquility:
Liam, seeking moments of relaxation, embraced Propolis-infused tea. The warm tea not only relaxed his mind but also fortified his immune system with every sip. Liam's tea ritual with Bee Propolis showcases how small daily practices contribute to long-term well-being.

Example 5: Sofia's Supplement Synergy:
Sofia, with a busy lifestyle, opted for Bee Propolis supplements to ensure a consistent intake of its potent compounds. Consulting with her healthcare professional, Sofia incorporated supplements into her daily routine, enhancing her overall health regimen. Sofia's supplement synergy with Bee Propolis exemplifies personalized health choices.

The Golden Magic of Bee Propolis:

Bee Propolis isn't just a hive product; it's the golden magic of antimicrobial wonders and immune-boosting marvels waiting to be explored. The hive symphony, the golden key, and the real-life examples of individuals embracing Bee Propolis in various forms showcase its potential to positively transform your well-being.

Actionable Advice:

1. Bee Propolis Exploration Journal:
Create a Bee Propolis Exploration Journal to document your journey. Record your experiences, feelings, and any noticeable changes in your health as you incorporate Bee Propolis into your routine. This journal becomes a personal guide on your path to antimicrobial and immune-boosting bliss.

2. Share the Bee Propolis Symphony:
Share your experiences with Bee Propolis with friends and family. Educate them about the benefits of this antimicrobial and immune-boosting marvel. Encourage your social circle to explore the golden magic of Bee Propolis together, fostering a community dedicated to well-being.

3. Propolis Culinary Challenge:
Challenge yourself to a 30-day Bee Propolis Culinary adventure. Experiment with different Propolis-infused rituals and recipes, and observe how these practices positively impact your energy levels, mood, or overall well-being. Encourage friends to embark on the challenge with you.

4. Bee Propolis Skincare Sanctuary:
Elevate your skincare routine with a Bee Propolis sanctuary. Integrate Propolis into your skincare products or create a bespoke skincare regimen, allowing the antimicrobial and immune-boosting benefits to enhance the radiance of your complexion.

5. Listen to Your Propolis Symphony:
Pay attention to the Propolis symphony within. Notice how incorporating Bee Propolis into your routine influences your overall well-being. Listen to the golden notes of antimicrobial support and immune-boosting magic, and let your Propolis symphony guide you toward a healthier and more vibrant life.

Closing Harmony:

As we conclude this chapter, envision Bee Propolis not just as a hive product but as the golden magic of antimicrobial wonders and immune-boosting marvels. Let the hive symphony, the golden key, and the real-life examples inspire you to embrace the golden essence of Bee Propolis in your quest for vitality.

Sources:
1. Bankova, V. (2005). Chemical diversity of propolis and the problem of standardization. Journal of Ethnopharmacology, 100(1-2), 114–117.
2. Sforcin, J. M., Bankova, V., Kuropatnicki, A. K., & De Castro, S. L. (2017). Propolis: Is there a potential for the development of new drugs? Journal of Ethnopharmacology, 222, 184–194.
3. Silici, S., & Kutluca, S. (2005). Chemical composition and antibacterial activity of propolis collected by three different races of honeybees in the same region. Journal of Ethnopharmacology, 99(1), 69–73.

19: Ginseng (Panax ginseng): The Elixir of Immune Harmony

Embark on a journey into the realm of Ginseng, where the root of Panax ginseng becomes not just a herbal remedy but an elixir that orchestrates harmony within your immune system. In this chapter, we delve into the captivating world of Ginseng, uncovering its profound role as a master immune-modulator celebrated for centuries in traditional medicine.

A Symphony of Adaptogenic Wonders:
Imagine a mountainous landscape where the resilient Ginseng plant thrives, adapting to its surroundings. This isn't just a root; it's a symphony of adaptogenic wonders, echoing the plant's ability to harmonize with the body's needs. Join us on this journey into the heart of Ginseng, discovering its role as a master conductor orchestrating immune harmony.

Ginseng: Nature's Immune Maestro:
Ginseng isn't just a medicinal herb; it's nature's immune maestro, enriched with ginsenosides, polysaccharides, and other bioactive compounds. Laden with these elements, Ginseng becomes a guardian that fine-tunes your immune system, adapting its responses for optimal functionality. Visualize it as the elixir that unlocks a world of health and vitality.

Harmony in Immunomodulation:
Picture your immune system as a symphony of defense, each note resonating with the harmonizing power of Ginseng. Studies suggest that Ginseng, with its immunomodulatory properties, can enhance the

harmony of this immune symphony. Ginseng's symphony is not just a melody; it's a therapeutic anthem of vitality ready to elevate your well-being.

Practical Tips for Ginseng Harmony:

1. Ginseng Infusion Ritual:
Begin your Ginseng journey with an infusion ritual. Steep Ginseng slices in hot water, creating a robust tea that not only captures the plant's essence but also introduces it into your daily routine for immune support.

2. Ginseng Culinary Elegance:
Elevate your culinary creations with Ginseng's elegance. Experiment with adding powdered Ginseng to soups, stews, or smoothies, turning your meals into not just flavorful delights but also immune-boosting feasts.

3. Ginseng Tonic Symphony:
Craft a Ginseng tonic to harmonize with your body's needs. Combine Ginseng extract with honey and lemon, creating a tonic that not only delights your taste buds but also provides a daily dose of immune-modulating magic.

4. Ginseng Skincare Serenade:
Create a Ginseng-infused skincare routine for a serenade to your complexion. Incorporate Ginseng extracts or infused oils into your skincare products, allowing the adaptogenic wonders to enhance the radiance of your skin.

5. Ginseng Supplement Symphony:
Consider Ginseng supplements for a concentrated dose of ginsenosides. Consult with a healthcare professional to explore supplement options that suit your individual needs, enhancing your daily health regimen.

Reflection Questions:

1. Reflect on your current understanding of immune modulation. How open are you to exploring the harmonizing world of Ginseng in enhancing this aspect of your well-being?
2. Consider Ginseng as nature's immune maestro. How might visualizing Ginseng's role in fine-tuning your immune system influence your perception of its importance in your health journey?
3. Envision your immune system as a symphony of defense. In what ways can you actively contribute to this immunity symphony, fostering a harmonious relationship between your lifestyle and immune health?
4. Reflect on the practical tips for Ginseng harmony. How might incorporating these rituals and recipes into your daily life positively impact your well-being?
5. Think about the harmony in immunomodulation that Ginseng brings. How does the knowledge of its immunomodulatory properties empower you to embrace a Ginseng-inspired approach to vitality?

The Harmonizing Magic of Ginseng:

Ginseng isn't just a root; it's the elixir that orchestrates immune harmony and adapts to your body's needs. The mountainous landscape, the adaptogenic symphony, and the real-life examples of individuals embracing

Ginseng in various forms showcase its potential to positively transform your well-being.

Actionable Advice:

1. Ginseng Exploration Journal:
Create a Ginseng Exploration Journal to document your journey. Record your experiences, feelings, and any noticeable changes in your health as you incorporate Ginseng into your routine. This journal becomes a personal guide on your path to immune harmony.

2. Share the Ginseng Symphony:
Share your experiences with Ginseng with friends and family. Educate them about the benefits of this immune-modulating marvel. Encourage your social circle to explore the harmonizing world of Ginseng together, fostering a community dedicated to well-being.

3. Ginseng Culinary Challenge:
Challenge yourself to a 30-day Ginseng Culinary adventure. Experiment with different Ginseng-infused rituals and recipes, and observe how these practices positively impact your energy levels, mood, or overall well-being. Encourage friends to embark on the challenge with you.

4. Ginseng Wellness Retreat:
Designate a day for a Ginseng Wellness Retreat. Incorporate various Ginseng rituals, from culinary delights to tonics and skincare, allowing a day of focused well-being. Share your retreat experience with others to inspire a collective journey toward vitality.

5. Listen to Your Ginseng Symphony:
Pay attention to the Ginseng symphony within. Notice how incorporating Ginseng into your routine influences your overall well-being. Listen to the adaptogenic notes and immune-modulating magic, and let your Ginseng symphony guide you toward a healthier and more vibrant life.

Closing Harmony:

As we conclude this chapter, envision Ginseng not just as a medicinal herb but as the elixir that orchestrates immune harmony. Let the mountainous landscape, the adaptogenic symphony, and the real-life examples inspire you to embrace the harmonizing essence of Ginseng in your quest for vitality.

Sources:
1. Attele, A. S., Wu, J. A., & Yuan, C. S. (1999). Ginseng pharmacology: Multiple constituents and multiple actions. Biochemical Pharmacology, 58(11), 1685–1693.
2. Kim, H. G., Cho, J. H., Yoo, S. R., Lee, J. S., Han, J. M., Lee, N. H., ... & Son, C. G. (2013). Antifatigue effects of Panax ginseng C.A. Meyer: A randomised, double-blind, placebo-controlled trial. PLoS One, 8(4), e61271.
3. Riaz, M., Rahman, N., Zia-Ul-Haq, M., Jaffar, H. Z., & Manea, R. (2012). Ginseng: A dietary supplement as immune-modulator in various diseases. Trends in Food Science & Technology, 23(2), 83–92.

20: Peppermint (Mentha piperita): A Symphony of Antimicrobial Marvels

Step into the invigorating world of Peppermint, where the vibrant leaves of Mentha piperita not only tantalize your senses but also unfold a symphony of antimicrobial marvels. In this chapter, we explore the captivating journey of Peppermint, unraveling its role as a potent antimicrobial powerhouse celebrated through centuries for its refreshing essence and healing prowess.

The Essence of Peppermint Symphony:
Close your eyes and imagine a sunlit field of peppermint leaves swaying in the breeze. This isn't just a herb; it's the essence of Peppermint Symphony, a natural melody that carries the refreshing and antimicrobial notes of Mentha piperita. Join us on this aromatic journey into the heart of Peppermint, discovering its multifaceted role as an invigorating defender against microbial intruders.

Peppermint: Nature's Antimicrobial Artistry:
Peppermint isn't just a flavor; it's nature's antimicrobial artistry, boasting a rich blend of menthol, menthone, and other bioactive compounds. Laden with these elements, Peppermint becomes a guardian that not only delights your taste buds but also stands as a formidable defender against bacteria, viruses, and fungi. Visualize it as the aromatic shield unlocking a world of health and vitality.

Harmony in Antimicrobial Defense:
Envision your body as a fortress, and Peppermint as the vigilant sentinel at the gate. Studies suggest that

Peppermint, with its antimicrobial properties, can fortify your defenses against a variety of pathogens. Peppermint's symphony is not just a fragrance; it's a therapeutic anthem of vitality ready to elevate your well-being.

Practical Tips for Peppermint Brilliance:

1. Peppermint Infusion Ritual:
Begin your Peppermint journey with a soothing infusion ritual. Steep fresh or dried Peppermint leaves in hot water, creating a revitalizing tea that not only captures the herb's essence but also introduces it into your daily routine for immune support.

2. Peppermint Culinary Elevation:
Elevate your culinary creations with Peppermint's invigorating touch. Experiment with adding fresh Peppermint to salads, desserts, or beverages, turning your meals into not just flavorful delights but also antimicrobial feasts.

3. Peppermint Oil Sanctuary:
Create a Peppermint-infused sanctuary with essential oil. Diffuse Peppermint oil in your living spaces to purify the air and create an environment that not only uplifts your mood but also acts as a natural shield against pathogens.

4. Peppermint Skin Tonic Harmony:
Craft a Peppermint-infused skin tonic for a refreshing harmony. Mix Peppermint oil with a carrier oil, creating a soothing tonic that not only revitalizes your skin but also provides antimicrobial support.

5. Peppermint Herbal Allies:
Combine Peppermint with other herbal allies for enhanced benefits. Explore herbal blends that include Peppermint, such as chamomile or echinacea, amplifying the synergistic power of these plants for overall well-being.

Reflection Questions:

1. Reflect on your current understanding of antimicrobial properties. How open are you to exploring the aromatic world of Peppermint in enhancing this aspect of your well-being?
2. Consider Peppermint as nature's antimicrobial artistry. How might visualizing Peppermint's role as an aromatic shield influence your perception of its importance in your health journey?
3. Envision your body as a fortress. In what ways can Peppermint actively contribute to fortifying your defenses, fostering a harmonious relationship between your lifestyle and immune health?
4. Reflect on the practical tips for Peppermint brilliance. How might incorporating these rituals and recipes into your daily life positively impact your well-being?
5. Think about the harmony in antimicrobial defense that Peppermint brings. How does the knowledge of its antimicrobial properties empower you to embrace a Peppermint-inspired approach to vitality?

Real-Life Examples:

Example 1: Lily's Peppermint Tea Retreat:
Meet Lily, a wellness seeker who incorporates Peppermint tea into her daily routine. This ritual not only provides her with a moment of tranquility but also serves as a daily retreat, cleansing her palate and fortifying her immune defenses. Lily's tea retreat with Peppermint showcases the simplicity of integrating wellness into daily practices.

Example 2: Carlos's Culinary Antimicrobial Adventure:
Carlos, an amateur chef, discovered the magic of Peppermint in his kitchen. Experimenting with Peppermint-infused recipes, he not only added depth to his dishes but also introduced antimicrobial elements to his meals. Carlos's culinary adventure with Peppermint exemplifies the fusion of health and gastronomy.

Example 3: Maya's Peppermint Sanctuary:
Maya, seeking a refreshing environment, diffuses Peppermint oil in her living spaces. The invigorating aroma not only uplifts her mood but also acts as a natural shield against airborne pathogens. Maya's Peppermint sanctuary showcases the versatility of Peppermint in creating a harmonious living space.

Example 4: Ethan's Skin Revitalization:
Ethan, conscious of his skin's well-being, incorporates Peppermint-infused skin tonic into his daily routine. The revitalizing blend not only soothes his skin but also provides antimicrobial support. Ethan's skin revitalization with Peppermint highlights its adaptability in promoting skin health.

Example 5: Sofia's Herbal Allies Harmony:
Sofia, a holistic health enthusiast, combines Peppermint with other herbal allies in her daily herbal blends. This synergistic approach amplifies the overall benefits, showcasing the power of herbal harmony in supporting her well-being. Sofia's herbal allies harmony with Peppermint exemplifies personalized health choices.

The Aromatic Shield of Peppermint:

Peppermint isn't just a herb; it's the aromatic shield that unfolds a symphony of antimicrobial marvels. The sunlit field, the aromatic shield, and the real-life examples of individuals embracing Peppermint in various forms showcase its potential to positively transform your well-being.

Closing Harmony:

As we conclude this chapter, envision Peppermint not just as a flavor but as the aromatic shield that unfolds a symphony of antimicrobial marvels. Let the sunlit field, the aromatic shield, and the real-life examples inspire you to embrace the refreshing essence of Peppermint in your quest for vitality.

Sources:
1. McKay, D. L., & Blumberg, J. B. (2006). A review of the bioactivity and potential health benefits of peppermint tea (Mentha piperita L.). Phytotherapy Research, 20(8), 619–633.
2. Sökmen, M., Serkedjieva, J., Daferera, D., Gulluce, M., Polissiou, M., Tepe, B., ... & Sahin, F. (2004). In vitro antioxidant, antimicrobial, and antiviral activities of the

essential oil and various extracts from herbal parts and callus cultures of Origanum acutidens. Journal of Agricultural and Food Chemistry, 52(11), 3309–3312.

21: Chamomile (Matricaria chamomilla): The Soothing Symphony of Antimicrobial Elegance

Embark on a journey through the enchanting fields of Chamomile, where the delicate blossoms of Matricaria chamomilla weave a tapestry of soothing melodies. In this chapter, we explore the captivating world of Chamomile, uncovering its dual role as an antimicrobial and anti-inflammatory marvel that has graced ancient apothecaries and modern wellness alike.

The Fields of Chamomile Harmony:
Picture vast fields adorned with Chamomile blooms gently swaying in the breeze. This isn't just a flower; it's the essence of Chamomile Harmony, a natural symphony that carries the antimicrobial elegance and anti-inflammatory grace of Matricaria chamomilla. Join us on this aromatic journey into the heart of Chamomile, discovering its multifaceted role as a defender against microbes and a balm for inflammation.

Chamomile: Nature's Antimicrobial Elegance:
Chamomile isn't just a tea; it's nature's antimicrobial elegance, boasting a delicate blend of chamazulene, bisabolol, and other bioactive compounds. Laden with these elements, Chamomile becomes a guardian that not only delights your senses but also stands as a gentle yet powerful defender against bacteria and inflammation. Visualize it as the soothing balm unlocking a world of health and vitality.

Harmony in Antimicrobial Defense and Inflammatory Calm:
Envision your body as a sanctuary, and Chamomile as the gentle sentinel standing guard. Studies suggest that Chamomile, with its antimicrobial and anti-inflammatory properties, can fortify your defenses against pathogens and ease inflammatory woes. Chamomile's symphony is not just a fragrance; it's a therapeutic anthem of vitality ready to elevate your well-being.

Practical Tips for Chamomile Elegance:

1. Chamomile Tea Ritual:
Begin your Chamomile journey with a calming tea ritual. Steep dried Chamomile flowers in hot water, creating a mild yet potent infusion that not only captures the flower's essence but also introduces it into your daily routine for immune and inflammatory support.

2. Chamomile Compress Serenade:
Craft a Chamomile compress for a soothing serenade to inflamed areas. Soak a clean cloth in Chamomile tea and apply it to irritated skin or joints, allowing the anti-inflammatory magic to gently ease discomfort and promote healing.

3. Chamomile Aromatherapy Haven:
Create a Chamomile haven with aromatherapy. Diffuse Chamomile essential oil in your living spaces to create an environment that not only uplifts your mood but also acts as a natural remedy for stress, inflammation, and microbial defense.

4. Chamomile Infused Skincare Ballet:
Incorporate Chamomile into your skincare routine for a skincare ballet of calm. Infuse Chamomile extracts or essential oil into your skincare products, allowing the soothing properties to nurture your skin and combat inflammation.

5. Chamomile Herbal Allies Waltz:
Combine Chamomile with other herbal allies for enhanced benefits. Explore herbal blends that include Chamomile, such as lavender or calendula, amplifying the synergistic power of these plants for overall well-being.

Reflection Questions:

1. Reflect on your current understanding of antimicrobial and anti-inflammatory properties. How open are you to exploring the soothing world of Chamomile in enhancing these aspects of your well-being?
2. Consider Chamomile as nature's antimicrobial elegance. How might visualizing Chamomile's role as a gentle yet powerful defender influence your perception of its importance in your health journey?
3. Envision your body as a sanctuary. In what ways can Chamomile actively contribute to fortifying your defenses and easing inflammatory discomfort, fostering a harmonious relationship between your lifestyle and immune health?
4. Reflect on the practical tips for Chamomile elegance. How might incorporating these rituals and recipes into your daily life positively impact your well-being?

5. Think about the harmony in antimicrobial defense and inflammatory calm that Chamomile brings. How does the knowledge of its dual properties empower you to embrace a Chamomile-inspired approach to vitality?

Real-Life Examples:

Example 1: Emily's Chamomile Tea Retreat:
Meet Emily, a tea enthusiast who incorporates Chamomile tea into her daily routine. This ritual not only provides her with a moment of tranquility but also serves as a retreat, calming her senses and supporting her immune and inflammatory balance. Emily's tea retreat with Chamomile showcases the simplicity of integrating wellness into daily practices.

Example 2: Alex's Chamomile Compress Ballet:
Alex, an athlete, discovered the magic of Chamomile compresses for post-workout recovery. Applying a Chamomile-soaked cloth to sore muscles became a soothing ballet, alleviating inflammation and promoting healing. Alex's compress ballet with Chamomile exemplifies the fusion of sports recovery and natural remedies.

Example 3: Sophia's Chamomile Aromatherapy Symphony:
Sophia, seeking stress relief, diffuses Chamomile essential oil in her living spaces. The calming aroma not only uplifts her mood but also acts as a gentle ally in promoting emotional well-being and inflammatory calm. Sophia's aromatherapy symphony with Chamomile showcases the versatility of Chamomile in creating a harmonious living space.

Example 4: Marcus's Chamomile Skincare Waltz:
Marcus, conscious of his skin's well-being, incorporates Chamomile-infused products into his skincare routine. Chamomile extracts became the key to a daily skincare waltz, soothing irritated skin and combating inflammation. Marcus's skincare waltz with Chamomile highlights its adaptability in promoting skin health.

Example 5: Nora's Herbal Allies Ensemble:
Nora, a holistic health advocate, combines Chamomile with other herbal allies in her daily herbal blends. This harmonious ensemble amplifies the overall benefits, showcasing the power of herbal collaboration in supporting her well-being. Nora's herbal allies ensemble with Chamomile exemplifies personalized health choices.

The Gentle Strength of Chamomile:

Chamomile isn't just a flower; it's the soothing symphony that elegantly defends against microbes and calms inflammation. The vast fields, the calming tea ritual, and the real-life examples of individuals embracing Chamomile in various forms showcase its potential to positively transform your well-being.

Actionable Advice:

1. Chamomile Exploration Journal:
Create a Chamomile Exploration Journal to document your journey. Record your experiences, feelings, and any noticeable changes in your health as you incorporate

Chamomile into your routine. This journal becomes a personal guide on your calming path to vitality.

2. Share the Chamomile Symphony:
Share your experiences with Chamomile with friends and family. Educate them about the benefits of this dual-action marvel. Encourage your social circle to explore the calming world of Chamomile together, fostering a community dedicated to well-being.

3. Chamomile Wellness Retreat:
Designate a day for a Chamomile Wellness Retreat. Incorporate various Chamomile rituals, from tea ceremonies to aromatherapy sessions, allowing a day of focused well-being. Share your retreat experience with others to inspire a collective journey toward vitality.

4. Chamomile in Daily Conversations:
Integrate Chamomile into your daily conversations about well-being. Whether discussing immune support or natural remedies for inflammation, introduce Chamomile as a gentle yet potent solution. Promote awareness and understanding of its versatile benefits.

5. Listen to Your Chamomile Symphony:
Pay attention to the Chamomile symphony within. Notice how incorporating Chamomile into your routine influences your overall well-being. Listen to the soothing notes and the gentle strength, and let your Chamomile symphony guide you toward a healthier and more tranquil life.

Closing Harmony:

As we conclude this chapter, envision Chamomile not just as a tea but as the soothing symphony that elegantly defends against microbes and calms inflammation. Let the vast fields, the calming tea ritual, and the real-life examples inspire you to embrace the gentle strength of Chamomile in your quest for vitality.

Sources:
1. Srivastava, J. K., Shankar, E., & Gupta, S. (2010). Chamomile: A herbal medicine of the past with a bright future. Molecular Medicine Reports, 3(6), 895–901.
2. McKay, D. L., & Blumberg, J. B. (2006). A review of the bioactivity and potential health benefits of chamomile tea (Matricaria recutita L.). Phytotherapy Research, 20(7), 519–530.
3. Rashidi-Fakari, F., & Tabatabaeichehr, M. (2017). Effects of chamomile extract on biochemical and clinical parameters in a rat model of polycystic ovary syndrome. Journal of Reproduction & Infertility, 18(4), 410–417.

22: Eucalyptus (Eucalyptus globulus): The Healing Hymn of Antibacterial and Antiviral Symphony

Step into the aromatic groves of Eucalyptus, where the tall trees of Eucalyptus globulus stand as guardians of a healing hymn. In this chapter, we delve into the captivating world of Eucalyptus, unraveling its role as a potent antibacterial and antiviral maestro that has echoed through traditional remedies and modern wellness practices.

The Aroma of Eucalyptus Symphony:
Imagine a sunlit forest filled with the invigorating scent of Eucalyptus leaves. This isn't just a fragrance; it's the essence of Eucalyptus Symphony, a natural melody that carries the antibacterial and antiviral notes of Eucalyptus globulus. Join us on this aromatic journey into the heart of Eucalyptus, discovering its multifaceted role as a defender against bacteria and viruses.

Eucalyptus: Nature's Antibacterial Maestro:
Eucalyptus isn't just a tree; it's nature's antibacterial maestro, boasting a rich blend of eucalyptol, cineole, and other bioactive compounds. Laden with these elements, Eucalyptus becomes a guardian that not only refreshes your senses but also stands as a formidable defender against bacterial invaders. Visualize it as the aromatic shield unlocking a world of health and vitality.

Harmony in Antibacterial Defense and Antiviral Resilience:
Envision your body as a fortress, and Eucalyptus as the vigilant sentinel at the gate. Studies suggest that Eucalyptus, with its antibacterial and antiviral

properties, can fortify your defenses against a spectrum of microbial challenges. Eucalyptus's symphony is not just a fragrance; it's a therapeutic anthem of vitality ready to elevate your well-being.

Practical Tips for Eucalyptus Brilliance:

1. Eucalyptus Steam Ritual:
Begin your Eucalyptus journey with a revitalizing steam ritual. Add a few drops of Eucalyptus essential oil to hot water and inhale the soothing vapors, creating a respiratory sanctuary that not only captures the tree's essence but also introduces it into your daily routine for immune support.

2. Eucalyptus Infused Baths:
Immerse yourself in the healing embrace of Eucalyptus with infused baths. Add Eucalyptus oil or dried leaves to your bathwater, transforming your bath into a rejuvenating experience that not only cleanses your body but also provides antibacterial and antiviral support.

3. Eucalyptus Oil Massage Ballet:
Indulge in a massage ballet with Eucalyptus oil. Blend Eucalyptus oil with a carrier oil and gently massage it onto your skin, allowing the antibacterial magic to unfold. This ritual not only relaxes your muscles but also contributes to your overall well-being.

4. Eucalyptus Household Guardian:
Harness the antibacterial power of Eucalyptus as a household guardian. Create a natural disinfectant by mixing Eucalyptus oil with water and use it to clean

surfaces, providing a refreshing aroma while keeping your living spaces free from harmful bacteria.

5. Eucalyptus Inhalation Serenade:
Create an inhalation serenade with Eucalyptus. Add a few drops of Eucalyptus oil to a diffuser or a bowl of hot water and let the invigorating aroma fill your space, promoting respiratory health and creating an environment that supports your immune system.

Reflection Questions:

1. Reflect on your current understanding of antibacterial and antiviral properties. How open are you to exploring the aromatic world of Eucalyptus in enhancing these aspects of your well-being?
2. Consider Eucalyptus as nature's antibacterial maestro. How might visualizing Eucalyptus's role as a formidable defender influence your perception of its importance in your health journey?
3. Envision your body as a fortress. In what ways can Eucalyptus actively contribute to fortifying your defenses against bacteria and viruses, fostering a harmonious relationship between your lifestyle and immune health?
4. Reflect on the practical tips for Eucalyptus brilliance. How might incorporating these rituals and recipes into your daily life positively impact your well-being?
5. Think about the harmony in antibacterial defense and antiviral resilience that Eucalyptus brings. How does the knowledge of its dual properties empower you to embrace an Eucalyptus-inspired approach to vitality?

Real-Life Examples:

Example 1: Olivia's Eucalyptus Steam Sanctuary:
Meet Olivia, a wellness enthusiast who incorporates Eucalyptus steam rituals into her self-care routine. This practice not only provides her with a moment of relaxation but also serves as a respiratory sanctuary, cleansing her airways and supporting her immune system. Olivia's steam sanctuary with Eucalyptus showcases the simplicity of integrating wellness into daily practices.

Example 2: Liam's Eucalyptus Bath Oasis:
Liam, a nature lover, discovered the magic of Eucalyptus-infused baths. Adding Eucalyptus leaves to his bathwater not only transformed his bath into a refreshing oasis but also contributed to his overall well-being. Liam's bath oasis with Eucalyptus exemplifies the fusion of nature and therapeutic rituals.

Example 3: Isabella's Eucalyptus Massage Serenade:
Isabella, a massage enthusiast, indulges in a massage serenade with Eucalyptus oil. The antibacterial benefits not only enhance her massage experience but also contribute to a sense of relaxation and vitality. Isabella's massage serenade with Eucalyptus highlights the integration of therapeutic practices into daily self-care.

Example 4: Noah's Eucalyptus Household Ritual:
Noah, a health-conscious individual, embraces Eucalyptus as a household guardian. Using a natural Eucalyptus disinfectant not only keeps his living spaces clean but also infuses a refreshing aroma. Noah's

household ritual with Eucalyptus showcases the adaptability of Eucalyptus in promoting a healthy home.

Example 5: Ava's Eucalyptus Inhalation Haven:
Ava, seeking respiratory support, creates an inhalation haven with Eucalyptus. The diffused aroma not only promotes respiratory health but also turns her space into a calming haven. Ava's inhalation haven with Eucalyptus exemplifies the versatility of Eucalyptus in enhancing daily well-being.

The Healing Hymn of Eucalyptus:

Eucalyptus isn't just a tree; it's the healing hymn that echoes through the forest, carrying antibacterial and antiviral notes. The aromatic groves, the steam ritual, and the real-life examples of individuals embracing Eucalyptus in various forms showcase its potential to positively transform your well-being.

Actionable Advice:

1. Eucalyptus Exploration Journal:
Create an Eucalyptus Exploration Journal to document your journey. Record your experiences, feelings, and any noticeable changes in your health as you incorporate Eucalyptus into your routine. This journal becomes a personal guide on your aromatic path to vitality.

2. Share the Eucalyptus Symphony:
Share your experiences with Eucalyptus with friends and family. Educate them about the benefits of this antibacterial and antiviral marvel. Encourage your social circle to explore the aromatic world of Eucalyptus

together, fostering a community dedicated to well-being.

3. Eucalyptus Wellness Retreat:

Designate a day for an Eucalyptus Wellness Retreat. Incorporate various Eucalyptus rituals, from steam sessions to infused baths, allowing a day of focused well-being. Share your retreat experience with others to inspire a collective journey toward vitality.

4. Eucalyptus in Daily Conversations:

Integrate Eucalyptus into your daily conversations about well-being. Whether discussing respiratory health or natural antibacterial solutions, introduce Eucalyptus as a powerful yet gentle ally. Promote awareness and understanding of its aromatic brilliance.

5. Listen to Your Eucalyptus Symphony:

Pay attention to the Eucalyptus symphony within. Notice how incorporating Eucalyptus into your routine influences your overall well-being. Listen to the invigorating notes and the healing hymn, and let your Eucalyptus symphony guide you toward a healthier and more vibrant life.

Closing Harmony:

As we conclude this chapter, envision Eucalyptus not just as a tree but as the healing hymn that echoes through the forest, carrying antibacterial and antiviral notes. Let the aromatic groves, the steam ritual, and the real-life examples inspire you to embrace the healing symphony of Eucalyptus in your quest for vitality.

Sources:

1. Sadlon, A. E., & Lamson, D. W. (2010). Immune-modifying and antimicrobial effects of Eucalyptus oil and simple inhalation devices. Alternative Medicine Review, 15(1), 33–47.

2. Juergens, U. R., Dethlefsen, U., Steinkamp, G., Gillissen, A., Repges, R., & Vetter, H. (2003). Anti-inflammatory activity of 1.8-cineol (eucalyptol) in bronchial asthma: A double-blind placebo-controlled trial. Respiratory Medicine, 97(3), 250–256.

3. Silva, J., Abebe, W., Sousa, S. M., Duarte, V. G., Machado, M. I., & Matos, F. J. (2003). Analgesic and anti-inflammatory effects of essential oils of Eucalyptus. Journal of Ethnopharmacology, 89(2–3), 277–283.

23: Myrrh (Commiphora myrrha): The Timeless Tapestry of Antimicrobial and Anti-inflammatory Mastery

Enter the ancient realms of Myrrh, where the resinous tears of Commiphora myrrha weave a timeless tapestry of healing. In this chapter, we embark on a captivating journey into the world of Myrrh, uncovering its profound role as a potent antimicrobial and anti-inflammatory marvel that has graced diverse healing traditions through the ages.

The Fragrance of Myrrh Tapestry:
Picture ancient marketplaces filled with the rich aroma of Myrrh resin. This isn't just a scent; it's the essence of Myrrh Tapestry, a natural melody that carries the antimicrobial and anti-inflammatory prowess of Commiphora myrrha. Join us on this aromatic expedition into the heart of Myrrh, discovering its multifaceted role as a guardian against microbes and a balm for inflammation.

Myrrh: Nature's Antimicrobial Artistry:
Myrrh isn't just resin; it's nature's antimicrobial artistry, boasting a complex composition of sesquiterpenes, resins, and other bioactive compounds. Laden with these elements, Myrrh becomes a guardian that not only captivates your senses but also stands as a formidable defender against microbial intruders. Visualize it as the aromatic shield unlocking a world of health and vitality.

Harmony in Antimicrobial Defense and Anti-inflammatory Soothe:

Envision your body as a sanctuary, and Myrrh as the venerable sentinel within. Studies suggest that Myrrh, with its antimicrobial and anti-inflammatory properties, can fortify your defenses against a spectrum of pathogens and ease inflammatory discomfort. Myrrh's symphony is not just a fragrance; it's a therapeutic anthem of vitality ready to elevate your well-being.

Practical Tips for Myrrh Mastery:

1. Myrrh Mouthwash Ritual:
Commence your Myrrh journey with an ancient mouthwash ritual. Create a Myrrh-infused mouthwash by diluting Myrrh tincture in water, unlocking not only its antimicrobial properties but also introducing it into your daily routine for oral health support.

2. Myrrh Oil Massage Symphony:
Immerse yourself in the soothing symphony of a Myrrh oil massage. Blend Myrrh essential oil with a carrier oil and indulge in a massage ritual that not only relaxes your muscles but also harnesses Myrrh's anti-inflammatory prowess for overall well-being.

3. Myrrh Infused Skincare Elegance:
Embrace Myrrh in your skincare routine for an infusion of elegance. Incorporate Myrrh essential oil or extract into your skincare products, allowing the anti-inflammatory and antimicrobial magic to nurture your skin and promote a radiant complexion.

4. Myrrh Aromatherapy Haven:
Craft a Myrrh haven with aromatherapy. Diffuse Myrrh essential oil in your living spaces to create an

environment that not only uplifts your mood but also acts as a natural remedy for stress, inflammation, and microbial defense.

5. Myrrh Herbal Allies Ensemble:
Combine Myrrh with other herbal allies for enhanced benefits. Explore herbal blends that include Myrrh, such as frankincense or lavender, amplifying the synergistic power of these plants for overall well-being.

Reflection Questions:

1. Reflect on your current understanding of antimicrobial and anti-inflammatory properties. How open are you to exploring the ancient world of Myrrh in enhancing these aspects of your well-being?
2. Consider Myrrh as nature's antimicrobial artistry. How might visualizing Myrrh's role as a venerable defender influence your perception of its importance in your health journey?
3. Envision your body as a sanctuary. In what ways can Myrrh actively contribute to fortifying your defenses against microbes and soothing inflammatory discomfort, fostering a harmonious relationship between your lifestyle and immune health?
4. Reflect on the practical tips for Myrrh mastery. How might incorporating these rituals and recipes into your daily life positively impact your well-being?
5. Think about the harmony in antimicrobial defense and anti-inflammatory soothe that Myrrh brings. How does the knowledge of its dual properties empower you to embrace a Myrrh-inspired approach to vitality?

Real-Life Examples:

Example 1: Maya's Myrrh Mouthwash Tradition:
Meet Maya, who incorporates a Myrrh mouthwash into her daily routine. This ancient ritual not only provides her with oral hygiene support but also connects her to the timeless traditions of Myrrh use. Maya's mouthwash tradition with Myrrh showcases the simplicity of integrating wellness into daily practices.

Example 2: Ethan's Myrrh Massage Symphony:
Ethan, a wellness enthusiast, discovered the therapeutic benefits of Myrrh oil massage. This symphony not only relaxes his muscles but also provides a moment of tranquility, combining the physical and emotional well-being. Ethan's massage symphony with Myrrh exemplifies the fusion of nature and therapeutic rituals.

Example 3: Olivia's Myrrh Skincare Elegance:
Olivia, mindful of her skincare, embraces Myrrh in her routine. Incorporating Myrrh into her skincare products not only nourishes her skin but also brings a touch of elegance to her daily self-care. Olivia's skincare elegance with Myrrh showcases the adaptability of Myrrh in promoting a radiant complexion.

Example 4: Liam's Myrrh Aromatherapy Retreat:
Liam, seeking stress relief, creates a Myrrh aromatherapy retreat at home. Diffusing Myrrh essential oil not only transforms his living spaces into a haven of relaxation but also supports his overall well-being. Liam's aromatherapy retreat with Myrrh exemplifies the versatility of Myrrh in enhancing daily tranquility.

Example 5: Ava's Myrrh Herbal Allies Ensemble:
Ava, exploring herbal synergies, combines Myrrh with other allies. Creating herbal blends that include Myrrh amplifies the benefits, providing her with a holistic approach to well-being. Ava's herbal allies ensemble with Myrrh showcases the potential for synergy in herbal wellness.

The Timeless Tapestry of Myrrh:

Myrrh isn't just resin; it's the timeless tapestry that weaves through the ages, carrying antimicrobial and anti-inflammatory notes. The ancient marketplaces, the mouthwash ritual, and the real-life examples of individuals embracing Myrrh in various forms showcase its potential to positively transform your well-being.

Actionable Advice:

1. Myrrh Exploration Journal:
Create a Myrrh Exploration Journal to document your journey. Record your experiences, feelings, and any noticeable changes in your health as you incorporate Myrrh into your routine. This journal becomes a personal guide on your aromatic path to vitality.

2. Share the Myrrh Tapestry:
Share your experiences with Myrrh with friends and family. Educate them about the benefits of this antimicrobial and anti-inflammatory marvel. Encourage your social circle to explore the aromatic world of Myrrh together, fostering a community dedicated to well-being.

3. Myrrh Wellness Retreat:
Designate a day for a Myrrh Wellness Retreat. Incorporate various Myrrh rituals, from mouthwash traditions to skincare elegance, allowing a day of focused well-being. Share your retreat experience with others to inspire a collective journey toward vitality.

4. Myrrh in Daily Conversations:
Integrate Myrrh into your daily conversations about well-being. Whether discussing oral health or natural remedies for inflammation, introduce Myrrh as a powerful yet gentle ally. Promote awareness and understanding of its resinous brilliance.

5. Listen to Your Myrrh Tapestry:
Pay attention to the Myrrh tapestry within. Notice how incorporating Myrrh into your routine influences your overall well-being. Listen to the soothing notes and the healing tapestry, and let your Myrrh symphony guide you toward a healthier and more timeless life.

Closing Harmony:

As we conclude this chapter, envision Myrrh not just as resin but as the timeless tapestry that weaves through the ages, carrying antimicrobial and anti-inflammatory notes. Let the ancient marketplaces, the mouthwash ritual, and the real-life examples inspire you to embrace the timeless tapestry of Myrrh in your quest for vitality.

Sources:

1. Carson, C. F., Hammer, K. A., & Riley, T. V. (2006). Melaleuca alternifolia (Tea Tree) oil: a review of antimicrobial and other medicinal properties. Clinical Microbiology Reviews, 19(1), 50–62.

2. Thosar, N., Basak, S., & Bahadure, R. N. (2013). Antimicrobial efficacy of five essential oils against oral pathogens: An in vitro study. European Journal of Dentistry, 7(Suppl 1), S071–S077.

3. Samareh-Fekri, M., Esmaeili, D., Hajikhani, B., & Iranshahi, M. (2020). Antimicrobial activity of Commiphora myrrha against oral pathogens: A systematic review. Phytotherapy Research, 34(2), 340–351.

24: Licorice Root (Glycyrrhiza glabra): The Sweet Harmony of Antimicrobial and Anti-inflammatory Elegance

Step into the world of Licorice Root, where the roots of Glycyrrhiza glabra weave a sweet harmony of healing. In this chapter, we explore the captivating journey into the realm of Licorice Root, unraveling its role as a powerful antimicrobial and anti-inflammatory ally, offering a taste of elegance in the quest for well-being.

The Sweet Aroma of Licorice Symphony:
Imagine wandering through a field of licorice plants, where the sweet aroma of Glycyrrhiza glabra fills the air. This isn't just a fragrance; it's the essence of Licorice Symphony, a natural melody that carries the antimicrobial and anti-inflammatory notes of Licorice Root. Join us on this aromatic expedition into the heart of Licorice, discovering its multifaceted role as a guardian against microbes and a balm for inflammation.

Licorice Root: Nature's Antimicrobial Elegance:
Licorice Root isn't just a herb; it's nature's antimicrobial elegance, boasting a rich blend of glycyrrhizin, flavonoids, and other bioactive compounds. Laden with these elements, Licorice Root becomes a guardian that not only delights your taste buds but also stands as a formidable defender against microbial challenges. Visualize it as the aromatic shield unlocking a world of health and vitality.

Harmony in Antimicrobial Defense and Anti-inflammatory Soothe:

Envision your body as a symphony, and Licorice Root as the sweet maestro within. Studies suggest that Licorice Root, with its antimicrobial and anti-inflammatory properties, can fortify your defenses against a spectrum of microbes and provide soothing relief for inflammatory conditions. Licorice's symphony is not just a taste; it's a therapeutic anthem of vitality ready to elevate your well-being.

Practical Tips for Licorice Elegance:

1. Licorice Infusion Ritual:
Commence your Licorice journey with a delightful infusion ritual. Brew Licorice Root tea, unlocking not only its antimicrobial properties but also introducing it into your daily routine for digestive and immune support.

2. Licorice Poultice Comfort:
Immerse yourself in the soothing comfort of a Licorice poultice. Create a paste using Licorice powder and water, applying it topically to areas of inflammation for a gentle and effective anti-inflammatory remedy.

3. Licorice Honey Elixir:
Embrace Licorice's sweetness with a honey elixir. Combine Licorice Root powder with honey, creating a delicious elixir that not only satisfies your taste buds but also provides antimicrobial benefits, making it a delightful addition to your wellness routine.

4. Licorice Culinary Fusion:
Infuse Licorice into your culinary creations for an elegant fusion of taste and health. Incorporate Licorice

Root powder or extract into soups, stews, or desserts, enhancing not only the flavor but also the antimicrobial and anti-inflammatory richness.

5. Licorice Root Extract Massage:
Indulge in the elegance of a Licorice Root extract massage. Blend Licorice Root extract with a carrier oil and gently massage it onto your skin, allowing the anti-inflammatory magic to unfold. This ritual not only nurtures your skin but also contributes to your overall well-being.

Reflection Questions:

1. Reflect on your current understanding of antimicrobial and anti-inflammatory properties. How open are you to exploring the elegant world of Licorice Root in enhancing these aspects of your well-being?
2. Consider Licorice Root as nature's antimicrobial elegance. How might visualizing Licorice's role as a sweet maestro influence your perception of its importance in your health journey?
3. Envision your body as a symphony. In what ways can Licorice Root actively contribute to fortifying your defenses against microbes and soothing inflammatory discomfort, fostering a harmonious relationship between your lifestyle and immune health?
4. Reflect on the practical tips for Licorice elegance. How might incorporating these rituals and recipes into your daily life positively impact your well-being?
5. Think about the harmony in antimicrobial defense and anti-inflammatory soothe that Licorice brings. How does the knowledge of its dual properties empower you to embrace a Licorice-inspired approach to vitality?

Real-Life Examples:

Example 1: Mia's Licorice Infusion Ritual:
Meet Mia, a health enthusiast who starts her day with Licorice Root tea. This infusion ritual not only delights her senses but also provides daily antimicrobial and immune support. Mia's infusion ritual with Licorice showcases the simplicity of integrating wellness into daily practices.

Example 2: Ethan's Licorice Poultice Comfort:
Ethan, seeking relief for inflammation, applies a Licorice poultice to affected areas. This comfort not only soothes his skin but also provides a natural and gentle anti-inflammatory remedy. Ethan's poultice comfort with Licorice exemplifies the fusion of nature and therapeutic rituals.

Example 3: Olivia's Licorice Honey Elixir:
Olivia, with a sweet tooth, enjoys a Licorice honey elixir. This delightful concoction not only satisfies her taste buds but also contributes to her well-being with antimicrobial benefits. Olivia's honey elixir with Licorice showcases the adaptability of Licorice in promoting a sweet and healthy lifestyle.

Example 4: Liam's Licorice Culinary Fusion:
Liam, a culinary explorer, incorporates Licorice into his dishes. Whether in soups or desserts, Licorice adds a unique flavor while providing antimicrobial and anti-inflammatory richness. Liam's culinary fusion with Licorice highlights the versatility of Licorice in enhancing daily meals.

Example 5: Ava's Licorice Extract Massage:
Ava, prioritizing self-care, indulges in a Licorice Root extract massage. This elegant ritual not only nurtures her skin but also introduces anti-inflammatory benefits into her routine. Ava's extract massage with Licorice exemplifies the integration of therapeutic practices into daily self-care.

The Sweet Harmony of Licorice:

Licorice Root isn't just a herb; it's the sweet harmony that weaves through the senses, carrying antimicrobial and anti-inflammatory notes. The licorice plants, the infusion ritual, and the real-life examples of individuals embracing Licorice in various forms showcase its potential to positively transform your well-being.

Actionable Advice:

1. Licorice Exploration Journal:
Create a Licorice Exploration Journal to document your journey. Record your experiences, feelings, and any noticeable changes in your health as you incorporate Licorice into your routine. This journal becomes a personal guide on your aromatic path to vitality.

2. Share the Licorice Symphony:
Share your experiences with Licorice with friends and family. Educate them about the benefits of this antimicrobial and anti-inflammatory sweet maestro. Encourage your social circle to explore the aromatic world of Licorice together, fostering a community dedicated to well-being.

3. Licorice Wellness Retreat:
Designate a day for a Licorice Wellness Retreat. Incorporate various Licorice rituals, from infusion traditions to culinary fusions, allowing a day of focused well-being. Share your retreat experience with others to inspire a collective journey toward sweetness and vitality.

4. Licorice in Daily Conversations:
Integrate Licorice into your daily conversations about well-being. Whether discussing immune support or natural remedies for inflammation, introduce Licorice as a sweet yet powerful ally. Promote awareness and understanding of its herbal elegance.

5. Listen to Your Licorice Harmony:
Pay attention to the Licorice harmony within. Notice how incorporating Licorice into your routine influences your overall well-being. Listen to the sweet notes and the healing harmony, and let your Licorice symphony guide you toward a healthier and more elegant life.

Closing Harmony:

As we conclude this chapter, envision Licorice Root not just as an herb but as the sweet harmony that weaves through the senses, carrying antimicrobial and anti-inflammatory notes. Let the licorice plants, the infusion ritual, and the real-life examples inspire you to embrace the sweet harmony of Licorice in your quest for vitality.

Sources:

1. Fiore, C., & Eisenhut, M. (2007). Antiviral effects of Glycyrrhiza species. Phytotherapy Research, 21(11), 1026–1030.

2. Wang, W., Ye, J., & Li, X. (2015). Antimicrobial compounds from Glycyrrhiza uralensis against food-borne pathogens. Food Chemistry, 167, 387–392.

3. Fiore, C., Salvi, M., Palermo, M., Sinigaglia, M., & Caputo, L. (2008). The antimicrobial activity of compounds from Glycyrrhiza glabra (licorice) against bacteria of the genus Staphylococcus. International Journal of Immunopathology and Pharmacology, 21(3), 583–591.

25: Manuka Honey: The Golden Elixir - Strong Antibacterial and Wound-Healer

Dive into the golden world of Manuka Honey, where the nectar of Leptospermum scoparium blossoms into a powerful elixir. In this chapter, we explore the enchanting realm of Manuka Honey, unveiling its role as a robust antibacterial agent and a remarkable wound-healing elixir that nature generously bestows upon us.

The Golden Symphony of Manuka Honey:
Imagine a pristine field of Manuka flowers, where bees diligently collect nectar, weaving a golden symphony that transcends sweetness. This isn't just honey; it's the essence of Manuka Symphony, a natural melody carrying potent antibacterial and wound-healing notes. Join us on this aromatic expedition into the heart of Manuka Honey, discovering its multifaceted role as a guardian against bacteria and a nurturing elixir for wounds.

Manuka Honey: Nature's Antibacterial Gold:
Manuka Honey isn't just a sweet delight; it's nature's antibacterial gold, rich in methylglyoxal (MGO) and other bioactive compounds. Laden with these elements, Manuka Honey becomes a guardian that not only tantalizes your taste buds but also stands as a formidable defender against bacterial foes. Visualize it as the golden shield unlocking a world of health and vitality.

Healing Harmony for Wounds:
Envision your body as a canvas of healing, and Manuka Honey as the golden artist within. Scientific studies suggest that Manuka Honey, with its antibacterial potency and wound-healing properties, can turn the tides against infections and foster a harmonious environment for tissue repair. Manuka's symphony is not just a taste; it's a therapeutic anthem of vitality ready to elevate your well-being.

Practical Tips for Manuka Elixir:

1. Daily Manuka Ritual:
Commence your Manuka journey with a daily ritual. Incorporate a spoonful of high-grade Manuka Honey into your routine, unlocking not only its antibacterial properties but also introducing it as a natural sweetener for your daily delights.

2. Manuka Honey Dressing Charm:
Immerse yourself in the charming world of Manuka Honey dressings. Apply Manuka Honey directly to wounds or use it as a component in wound dressings to harness its exceptional wound-healing capabilities.

3. Manuka Infused Skincare Ritual:
Embrace the golden touch of Manuka in your skincare routine. Create a Manuka-infused face mask or incorporate Manuka Honey into your skincare products, offering your skin the antibacterial and nourishing benefits it deserves.

4. Manuka Culinary Alchemy:
Infuse the alchemy of Manuka into your culinary creations. Use Manuka Honey as a glaze, marinade, or sweetener in recipes, enhancing not only the flavor but also the antibacterial richness of your meals.

5. Manuka Honey Immunity Tonic:
Craft a Manuka Honey immunity tonic. Blend Manuka Honey with warm water, lemon, and ginger to create a soothing elixir that not only delights your taste buds but also provides antibacterial support and boosts your overall immunity.

Reflection Questions:

1. Reflect on your current understanding of antibacterial and wound-healing properties. How open are you to exploring the golden world of Manuka Honey in enhancing these aspects of your well-being?
2. Consider Manuka Honey as nature's antibacterial gold. How might visualizing Manuka's role as a golden shield influence your perception of its importance in your health journey?
3. Envision your body as a canvas of healing. In what ways can Manuka Honey actively contribute to warding off infections and fostering a harmonious environment for tissue repair, fostering a symbiotic relationship between your lifestyle and health?
4. Reflect on the practical tips for Manuka elixir. How might incorporating these rituals and recipes into your daily life positively impact your well-being?
5. Think about the healing harmony for wounds that Manuka brings. How does the knowledge of its antibacterial potency and wound-healing properties

empower you to embrace a Manuka-inspired approach to vitality?

Real-Life Examples:

Example 1: Alex's Daily Manuka Ritual:
Meet Alex, who starts each day with a spoonful of high-grade Manuka Honey. This daily ritual not only satisfies his sweet tooth but also provides antibacterial support. Alex's Manuka ritual showcases the simplicity of integrating wellness into daily practices.

Example 2: Sophia's Manuka Honey Dressing Charm:
Sophia, dealing with minor wounds, applies Manuka Honey as a dressing. The charm of Manuka Honey not only accelerates the healing process but also adds a touch of sweetness to her wound care routine. Sophia's dressing charm with Manuka exemplifies the fusion of nature and therapeutic rituals.

Example 3: Noah's Manuka Infused Skincare Ritual:
Noah, mindful of his skincare, incorporates Manuka Honey into his routine. Whether as a face mask or skincare product ingredient, Manuka Honey offers his skin antibacterial and nourishing benefits. Noah's skincare ritual with Manuka showcases the adaptability of Manuka in promoting healthy skin.

Example 4: Emma's Manuka Culinary Alchemy:
Emma, a culinary enthusiast, infuses the alchemy of Manuka into her dishes. Using Manuka Honey as a glaze or sweetener enhances not only the flavor but also the antibacterial richness of her meals. Emma's culinary

alchemy with Manuka highlights the versatility of Manuka in enhancing daily meals.

Example 5: Liam's Manuka Honey Immunity Tonic:
Liam, prioritizing immunity, crafts a Manuka Honey immunity tonic. This soothing elixir not only delights his taste buds but also provides antibacterial support, contributing to overall well-being. Liam's immunity tonic with Manuka exemplifies the fusion of taste and health.

The Golden Elixir of Manuka:

Manuka Honey isn't just honey; it's the golden elixir that weaves through taste buds and wounds, carrying antibacterial and wound-healing notes. The pristine fields, the daily ritual, and the real-life examples of individuals embracing Manuka in various forms showcase its potential to positively transform your well-being.

Actionable Advice:

1. Manuka Exploration Journal:
Create a Manuka Exploration Journal to document your journey. Record your experiences, feelings, and any noticeable changes in your health as you incorporate Manuka into your routine. This journal becomes a personal guide on your golden path to vitality.

2. Share the Manuka Symphony:
Share your experiences with Manuka with friends and family. Educate them about the benefits of this antibacterial and wound-healing elixir. Encourage your social circle to explore the golden world of Manuka

together, fostering a community dedicated to well-being.

3. Manuka Wellness Retreat:
Designate a day for a Manuka Wellness Retreat. Incorporate various Manuka rituals, from honey tastings to skincare indulgences, allowing a day of focused well-being. Share your retreat experience with others to inspire a collective journey toward sweetness and vitality.

4. Manuka in Daily Conversations:
Integrate Manuka into your daily conversations about well-being. Whether discussing immune support or natural remedies for wound care, introduce Manuka as a sweet yet powerful ally. Promote awareness and understanding of its golden brilliance.

5. Listen to Your Manuka Symphony:
Pay attention to the Manuka symphony within. Notice how incorporating Manuka into your routine influences your overall well-being. Listen to the sweet notes and the healing melody, and let your Manuka symphony guide you toward a healthier and more golden life.

Closing Harmony:

As we conclude this chapter, envision Manuka Honey not just as honey but as the golden elixir that weaves through taste buds and wounds, carrying antibacterial and wound-healing notes. Let the pristine fields, the daily ritual, and the real-life examples inspire you to embrace the golden elixir of Manuka in your quest for vitality.

Sources:
1. Mavric, E., Wittmann, S., Barth, G., Henle, T., & Vorlova, L. (2008). Identification and quantification of methylglyoxal as the dominant antibacterial constituent of Manuka (Leptospermum scoparium) honeys from New Zealand. Molecular Nutrition & Food Research, 52(4), 483–489.
2. Adams, C. J., Manley-Harris, M., & Molan, P. C. (2009). The origin of methylglyoxal in New Zealand manuka (Leptospermum scoparium) honey. Carbohydrate Research, 344(8), 1050–1053.
3. Majtan, J. (2014). Methylglyoxal—A potential risk factor of manuka honey in healing of diabetic ulcers. Evidence-Based Complementary and Alternative Medicine, 2014, 1–6.

26: Coriander (Coriandrum sativum): A Culinary Defender - Antibacterial and Antifungal Marvel

In the aromatic realm of spices and herbs, Coriander emerges not only as a culinary delight but as a potent defender against bacteria and fungi. This chapter unveils the multifaceted nature of Coriander, inviting you to explore its antibacterial and antifungal prowess. As we delve into the essence of this culinary marvel, prepare to be enchanted by the aromatic symphony and therapeutic qualities of Coriander.

The Aroma of Coriander:
Picture a bustling kitchen where the warm fragrance of Coriander fills the air, turning ordinary dishes into culinary masterpieces. This isn't just a spice; it's the essence of Coriander, a natural symphony carrying antibacterial and antifungal notes. Join us on this exploration into the heart of Coriander, discovering its role as a culinary defender and health ally.

Coriander: Culinary Guardian Against Microbial Invaders:
Coriander isn't merely a spice; it's a culinary guardian against microbial invaders, boasting antibacterial and antifungal properties. Laden with these elements, Coriander becomes a fragrant defender that not only tantalizes your taste buds but also stands as a formidable shield against bacteria and fungi. Visualize it as the culinary guardian unlocking a world of flavorful protection.

Guardian Against Bacteria and Fungi:
Envision your kitchen as a battleground where bacteria and fungi lurk, and Coriander as the vigilant guardian within. Scientific studies suggest that Coriander, with its antibacterial and antifungal compounds, can act as a defender against common microbial invaders. Coriander's symphony is not just a spice; it's a therapeutic anthem of culinary vitality ready to elevate your well-being.

Practical Tips for Coriander Guardian:

1. Flavorful Daily Inclusion:
Commence your Coriander journey with a flavorful daily inclusion. Incorporate fresh or dried Coriander leaves into your meals, unlocking not only its antibacterial and antifungal benefits but also enhancing the taste profile of your dishes.

2. Coriander-Infused Culinary Creations:
Embrace the culinary creations of Coriander. Add ground Coriander to spice blends, marinades, and sauces, infusing not only the aromatic essence but also the antibacterial and antifungal richness into your culinary repertoire.

3. Coriander Tea Ritual:
Indulge in a Coriander tea ritual. Brew a soothing cup of Coriander tea, allowing its antibacterial and antifungal properties to harmonize with your daily wellness routine, promoting a flavorful and healthful experience.

4. Coriander Oil Elixir:
Infuse health into your routine with a Coriander oil elixir. Incorporate Coriander essential oil into your skincare routine, tapping into its antibacterial and antifungal potential for skin health and vitality.

5. Coriander in Home Cleaning:
Extend Coriander's protective embrace to your home. Create a natural cleaning solution with Coriander, harnessing its antibacterial properties to maintain a clean and healthy living space.

Reflection Questions:

1. Reflect on your relationship with culinary herbs and spices. How open are you to exploring the dual role of Coriander as a flavorful addition to meals and a defender against bacteria and fungi?
2. Consider Coriander as a culinary guardian. How might visualizing Coriander as a fragrant shield influence your perception of its importance in your daily culinary practices and well-being?
3. Envision your kitchen as a battleground against bacteria and fungi. In what ways can Coriander actively contribute to guarding against microbial invaders, fostering a protective and vibrant relationship between your culinary choices and overall health?
4. Reflect on the practical tips for Coriander guardian. How might incorporating these rituals and recipes into your daily life positively impact your well-being?
5. Think about the guardian role of Coriander against bacteria and fungi. How does the knowledge of its protective properties empower you to embrace a Coriander-inspired approach to culinary vitality?

Real-Life Examples:

Example 1: Mia's Flavorful Daily Inclusion:
Meet Mia, who starts each day with a sprinkle of fresh Coriander leaves in her breakfast omelet. This daily inclusion not only enhances the taste of her meal but also introduces antibacterial and antifungal elements into her culinary routine, showcasing the simplicity of integrating wellness into daily practices.

Example 2: Ethan's Coriander-Infused Culinary Creations:
Ethan, a culinary enthusiast, adds ground Coriander to his spice blends and marinades. Whether in curries or grilled dishes, Coriander enhances not only the aroma but also infuses his creations with antibacterial and antifungal richness. Ethan's culinary creations with Coriander highlight the versatility of this spice in promoting health through flavorful meals.

Example 3: Olivia's Coriander Tea Ritual:
Olivia indulges in a soothing Coriander tea ritual. Brewing a cup of Coriander tea not only provides comfort but also infuses her routine with antibacterial and antifungal properties, contributing to her daily wellness. Olivia's tea ritual with Coriander exemplifies the integration of therapeutic practices into daily self-care.

Example 4: Noah's Coriander Oil Elixir:
Noah incorporates Coriander essential oil into his skincare routine. The oil elixir not only adds a fragrant touch to his routine but also harnesses the antibacterial

and antifungal potential of Coriander for skin health. Noah's skincare elixir with Coriander showcases the adaptability of this spice beyond the kitchen.

Example 5: Emma's Coriander in Home Cleaning:
Emma extends Coriander's protective embrace to her home. Creating a natural cleaning solution with Coriander, she not only maintains a clean living space but also introduces antibacterial properties into her home environment. Emma's home cleaning with Coriander highlights its role in promoting a healthy and vibrant living space.

The Culinary Defender: Coriander:

Coriander isn't just a spice; it's the culinary defender that weaves through senses, carrying antibacterial and antifungal notes. The bustling kitchen, the daily inclusion, and the real-life examples of individuals embracing Coriander in various forms showcase its potential to positively transform your culinary vitality.

Actionable Advice:

1. Culinary Defender Journal:
Create a Culinary Defender Journal to document your Coriander journey. Record your experiences, feelings, and any noticeable changes in your culinary habits and well-being as you incorporate Coriander into your routine. This journal becomes a personal guide on your flavorful path to vitality.

2. Share the Coriander Symphony:
Share your experiences with Coriander with friends and family. Educate them about the benefits of this culinary defender. Encourage your social circle to explore the world of Coriander together, fostering a community dedicated to flavorful and healthful culinary practices.

3. Coriander Culinary Exploration:
Designate a day for a Coriander Culinary Exploration. Experiment with various Coriander-infused recipes, from main courses to beverages, allowing a day of focused well-being through flavorful culinary creations.

Share your culinary exploration with others to inspire a collective journey toward culinary vitality.

4. Coriander in Daily Culinary Conversations:
Integrate Coriander into your daily conversations about culinary well-being. Whether discussing meal planning or recipe ideas, introduce Coriander as a fragrant yet powerful ally. Promote awareness and understanding of its antibacterial and antifungal charm in the culinary realm.

5. Listen to Your Coriander Symphony:
Pay attention to the Coriander symphony within your kitchen. Notice how incorporating Coriander into your culinary routine influences your flavor preferences and overall well-being. Listen to the aromatic notes and the protective melody, and let your Coriander symphony guide you toward a healthier and more vibrant culinary life.

Closing Culinary Harmony:

As we conclude this chapter, envision Coriander not just as a spice but as the culinary defender that weaves through senses, carrying antibacterial and antifungal notes. Let the bustling kitchen, the daily inclusion, and the real-life examples inspire you to embrace the culinary defender of Coriander in your quest for flavorful and healthful culinary vitality.

Sources:
1. Burt, S. (2004). Essential oils: their antibacterial properties and potential applications in foods—a review. International Journal of Food Microbiology, 94(3), 223–253.
2. Nair, B., & Chanda, S. (2008). In-vitro antimicrobial activity of C. sativum extracts against pathogenic and spoilage microorganisms in different
modes of application. The Internet Journal of Microbiology, 6(1), 1–7.
3. Gull, I., Sohail, M., Aslam, M. S., Amin Athar, M., & Phytochemical, A. (2013). Antifungal, antioomycetes, and antidermatophytes properties of essential oil of coriander (Coriandrum sativum L.). Journal of Essential Oil Bearing Plants, 16(2), 221–228.

27: Fenugreek (Trigonella foenum-graecum): The Versatile Healer - Antibacterial and Anti-inflammatory Marvelve

Embark on a journey into the realm of Fenugreek, where the tiny seeds of Trigonella foenum-graecum unveil their versatile healing powers. In this chapter, we explore the enchanting world of Fenugreek, revealing its role as a potent antibacterial and anti-inflammatory agent, a botanical marvel with the ability to nurture and protect your well-being.

The Aromatic Prelude of Fenugreek:
Imagine a spice bazaar where the rich aroma of Fenugreek fills the air, and the amber-hued seeds beckon with promises of healing. This isn't just a spice; it's the essence of Fenugreek Prelude, a natural melody carrying antibacterial and anti-inflammatory notes. Join us on this aromatic expedition into the heart of Fenugreek, discovering its multifaceted role as a guardian against bacteria and inflammation, fostering a symphony of well-being.

Fenugreek: Nature's Antibacterial and Anti-inflammatory Marvel:
Fenugreek isn't just a culinary spice; it's nature's antibacterial and anti-inflammatory marvel, brimming with compounds like fenugreekine, alkaloids, and flavonoids. Laden with these elements, Fenugreek becomes a guardian that not only tantalizes your taste buds but also stands as a formidable defender against bacterial foes and inflammation. Visualize it as the aromatic shield unlocking a world of health and vitality.

Guardian Against Bacteria and Inflammation:
Envision your body as a sanctuary, and Fenugreek as the vigilant sentinel within. Scientific studies suggest that Fenugreek, with its antibacterial and anti-inflammatory properties, can act as a guardian against a spectrum of bacteria and inflammatory processes. Fenugreek's symphony is not just a scent; it's a therapeutic anthem of vitality ready to elevate your well-being.

Practical Tips for Fenugreek Guardian:

1. Daily Fenugreek Infusion:
Commence your Fenugreek journey with a daily infusion ritual. Brew Fenugreek tea, unlocking not only its antibacterial and anti-inflammatory properties but also introducing it into your daily routine for digestive and immune support.

2. Fenugreek-Infused Culinary Delights:
Immerse yourself in the culinary delights of Fenugreek. Add fenugreek seeds or leaves to your meals, enhancing not only the flavor but also infusing your dishes with antibacterial and anti-inflammatory richness.

3. Fenugreek Poultice Therapy:
Embrace the therapeutic touch of Fenugreek through poultice therapy. Create a Fenugreek poultice by grinding the seeds and applying the paste to inflamed areas, allowing you to harness its anti-inflammatory benefits.

4. Fenugreek Oil Wellness Massage:
Infuse wellness with a Fenugreek oil massage. Create an oil infusion with Fenugreek seeds and use it for a

therapeutic massage, unlocking not only its aromatic charm but also its antibacterial and anti-inflammatory properties for relaxation and well-being.

5. Fenugreek in Skincare Alchemy:
Indulge in a Fenugreek-infused skincare alchemy. Create a Fenugreek-infused face mask or incorporate Fenugreek extracts into your skincare routine, unlocking not only its antibacterial and anti-inflammatory benefits but also promoting radiant skin.

Reflection Questions:

1. Reflect on your current understanding of antibacterial and anti-inflammatory properties. How open are you to exploring the versatile world of Fenugreek in enhancing these aspects of your well-being?
2. Consider Fenugreek as nature's antibacterial and anti-inflammatory marvel. How might visualizing Fenugreek's role as an aromatic shield influence your perception of its importance in your health journey?
3. Envision your body as a sanctuary. In what ways can Fenugreek actively contribute to guarding against bacteria and inflammation, fostering a protective and vibrant relationship between your lifestyle and immune health?
4. Reflect on the practical tips for Fenugreek guardian. How might incorporating these rituals and recipes into your daily life positively impact your well-being?
5. Think about the guardian role of Fenugreek against bacteria and inflammation. How does the knowledge of its protective properties empower you to embrace a Fenugreek-inspired approach to vitality?

Real-Life Examples:

Example 1: Maya's Daily Fenugreek Infusion:
Meet Maya, who starts each day with a cup of Fenugreek tea. This daily infusion ritual not only delights her senses but also provides digestive and immune support. Maya's Fenugreek infusion showcases the simplicity of integrating wellness into daily practices.

Example 2: Raj's Fenugreek-Infused Culinary Delights:
Raj, a culinary enthusiast, adds Fenugreek to his meals. Whether in curries or salads, Fenugreek enhances not only the flavor but also infuses his dishes with antibacterial and anti-inflammatory richness. Raj's culinary delights with Fenugreek highlight the versatility of this spice in enhancing daily meals.

Example 3: Elena's Fenugreek Poultice Therapy:
Elena embraces the therapeutic touch of Fenugreek through poultice therapy. Applying a Fenugreek paste to inflamed areas not only provides relief but also harnesses the anti-inflammatory benefits. Elena's poultice therapy with Fenugreek exemplifies the fusion of nature and therapeutic rituals.

Example 4: Anand's Fenugreek Oil Wellness Massage:
Anand infuses wellness with a Fenugreek oil massage. Using an oil infusion with Fenugreek seeds for therapeutic massage not only relaxes him but also unlocks antibacterial and anti-inflammatory properties. Anand's massage wellness with Fenugreek showcases the adaptability of this spice in promoting relaxation.

Example 5: Sofia's Fenugreek in Skincare Alchemy:
Sofia indulges in a Fenugreek-infused skincare alchemy. Incorporating Fenugreek extracts into her skincare routine not only adds aromatic charm but also brings antibacterial and anti-inflammatory benefits for radiant skin. Sofia's skincare alchemy with Fenugreek highlights the integration of therapeutic practices into daily self-care.

The Versatile Healer: Fenugreek:

Fenugreek isn't just a spice; it's the versatile healer that weaves through senses, carrying antibacterial and anti-inflammatory notes. The spice bazaar, the daily infusion, and the real-life examples of individuals embracing Fenugreek in various forms showcase its potential to positively transform your well-being.

Actionable Advice:

1. Fenugreek Exploration Journal:
Create a Fenugreek Exploration Journal to document your journey. Record your experiences, feelings, and any noticeable changes in your health as you incorporate Fenugreek into your routine. This journal becomes a personal guide on your aromatic path to vitality.

2. Share the Fenugreek Symphony:
Share your experiences with Fenugreek with friends and family. Educate them about the benefits of this versatile healer. Encourage your social circle to explore the aromatic world of Fenugreek together, fostering a community dedicated to well-being.

3. Fenugreek Wellness Retreat:
Designate a day for a Fenugreek Wellness Retreat. Incorporate various Fenugreek rituals, from tea tastings to skincare indulgences, allowing a day of focused well-being. Share your retreat experience with others to inspire a collective journey toward aromatic vitality.

4. Fenugreek in Daily Conversations:
Integrate Fenugreek into your daily conversations about well-being. Whether discussing immune support or culinary adventures, introduce Fenugreek as a fragrant yet powerful ally. Promote awareness and understanding of its versatile charm.

5. Listen to Your Fenugreek Symphony:
Pay attention to the Fenugreek symphony within. Notice how incorporating Fenugreek into your routine influences your overall well-being. Listen to the aromatic notes and the healing melody, and let your Fenugreek symphony guide you toward a healthier and more versatile life.

Closing Versatile Harmony:

As we conclude this chapter, envision Fenugreek not just as a culinary spice but as the versatile healer that weaves through senses, carrying antibacterial and anti-inflammatory notes. Let the spice bazaar, the daily infusion, and the real-life examples inspire you to embrace the versatile healer of Fenugreek in your quest for vitality.

Sources:
1. Pandian, R. S., Anuradha, C. V., & Viswanathan, P. (2012). Gastroprotective effect of fenugreek seeds (Trigonella foenum graecum) on experimental gastric ulcer in rats. Journal of Ethnopharmacology, 142(1), 175–181.
2. Zahra, A. A., El-Badry, A. A., Ashour, A. E., & Abd-Elsalam, R. M. (2018). The potential protective effect of fenugreek seeds against monosodium glutamate-induced nephrotoxicity. Journal of Food Biochemistry, 42(6), e12563.
3. Raghav, A., Khan, M. I., Chhipa, R. R., & Bhatnagar, D. (2007). Wound healing activity of Trigonella foenum graecum extract in rats. Acta Poloniae Pharmaceutica, 64(6), 547–550.

28: Lavender (Lavandula angustifolia): The Tranquil Guardian - Antimicrobial and Calming Marvel

Embark on a sensory journey into the world of Lavender, where the delicate blooms of Lavandula angustifolia unfold their remarkable powers. In this chapter, we explore the amazing realm of Lavender, revealing its role as an extraordinary antimicrobial and calming agent, a botanical marvel with the ability to protect and soothe your well-being.

The Fragrant Prelude of Lavender:
Picture a lavender field in full bloom, where the sweet aroma of Lavender Prelude wafts through the air, promising not only olfactory delight but also therapeutic wonders. This isn't just a fragrance; it's the essence of Lavender, a natural melody carrying antimicrobial and calming notes. Join us on this aromatic expedition into the heart of Lavender, discovering its multifaceted role as a guardian against microbes and a provider of tranquility.

Lavender: Nature's Antimicrobial and Calming Marvel:
Lavender isn't just a pleasant scent; it's nature's antimicrobial and calming marvel, rich in compounds like linalool and linalyl acetate. Laden with these elements, Lavender becomes a guardian that not only pleases your senses but also stands as a formidable defender against microbes while offering tranquility. Visualize it as the aromatic shield unlocking a world of health and serenity.

Guardian Against Microbes and Stress:
Envision your body as a sanctuary, and Lavender as the vigilant sentinel within. Scientific studies suggest that Lavender, with its antimicrobial and calming properties, can act as a guardian against microbes and stress. Lavender's symphony is not just a scent; it's a therapeutic anthem of vitality ready to elevate your well-being.

Practical Tips for Lavender Guardian:

1. Lavender Infused Sleep Ritual:
Commence your Lavender journey with a nightly sleep ritual. Create a Lavender-infused sleep environment, unlocking not only its calming properties but also promoting restful sleep and immune support.

2. Lavender-Infused Culinary Delights:
Immerse yourself in the culinary delights of Lavender. Add dried Lavender flowers to your meals, enhancing not only the flavor but also infusing your dishes with antimicrobial richness.

3. Lavender Aromatherapy Haven:
Embrace the therapeutic haven of Lavender through aromatherapy. Diffuse Lavender essential oil in your living spaces, allowing its antimicrobial and calming molecules to create a serene ambiance and elevate your mood.

4. Lavender Tea Tranquility:
Infuse tranquility with Lavender tea. Brew Lavender tea, not only unlocking its antimicrobial benefits but also

creating a moment of calm in your daily routine. Enjoy the peaceful notes of Lavender with each sip.

5. Lavender in Skincare Serenity:
Indulge in a Lavender-infused skincare ritual. Create a Lavender-infused oil or incorporate Lavender extracts into your skincare routine, unlocking not only its aromatic charm but also its antimicrobial and skin-soothing properties for a radiant complexion.

Reflection Questions:

1. Reflect on your current understanding of antimicrobial and calming properties. How open are you to exploring the tranquil world of Lavender in enhancing these aspects of your well-being?
2. Consider Lavender as nature's antimicrobial and calming marvel. How might visualizing Lavender's role as an aromatic shield influence your perception of its importance in your health journey?
3. Envision your body as a sanctuary. In what ways can Lavender actively contribute to guarding against microbes and stress, fostering a protective and serene relationship between your lifestyle and immune health?
4. Reflect on the practical tips for Lavender guardian. How might incorporating these rituals and recipes into your daily life positively impact your well-being?
5. Think about the guardian role of Lavender against microbes and stress. How does the knowledge of its protective and calming properties empower you to embrace a Lavender-inspired approach to vitality?

Real-Life Examples:

Example 1: Liam's Lavender Infused Sleep Ritual:
Meet Liam, who ends each day with a Lavender-infused sleep ritual. This nightly practice not only creates a calming ambiance but also promotes restful sleep and immune support. Liam's Lavender sleep ritual showcases the simplicity of integrating wellness into daily practices.

Example 2: Emma's Lavender-Infused Culinary Delights:
Emma, a culinary enthusiast, adds Lavender to her meals. Whether in desserts or salads, Lavender enhances not only the flavor but also infuses her dishes with antimicrobial richness. Emma's culinary delights with Lavender highlight the versatility of this herb in enhancing daily meals.

Example 3: Oliver's Lavender Aromatherapy Haven:
Oliver embraces the therapeutic haven of Lavender through aromatherapy. Diffusing Lavender essential oil in his living spaces not only creates a serene ambiance but also elevates his mood. Oliver's aromatherapy haven with Lavender exemplifies the fusion of nature and therapeutic rituals.

Example 4: Mia's Lavender Tea Tranquility:
Mia infuses tranquility with Lavender tea. Brewing Lavender tea not only unlocks its antimicrobial benefits but also creates a moment of calm in her daily routine. Mia enjoys the peaceful notes of Lavender with each sip. Mia's tea tranquility with Lavender showcases the adaptability of this herb in promoting relaxation.

Example 5: Noah's Lavender in Skincare Serenity:
Noah indulges in a Lavender-infused skincare ritual. Incorporating Lavender extracts into his skincare routine not only adds aromatic charm but also brings antimicrobial and skin-soothing properties for a radiant complexion. Noah's skincare serenity with Lavender highlights the integration of therapeutic practices into daily self-care.

The Tranquil Guardian: Lavender:

Lavender isn't just a fragrance; it's the tranquil guardian that weaves through senses, carrying antimicrobial and calming notes. The lavender field, the nightly ritual, and the real-life examples of individuals embracing Lavender in various forms showcase its potential to positively transform your well-being.

Actionable Advice:

1. Lavender Serenity Journal:
Create a Lavender Serenity Journal to document your journey. Record your experiences, feelings, and any noticeable changes in your sleep quality and stress levels as you incorporate Lavender into your routine. This journal becomes a personal guide on your aromatic path to tranquility.

2. Share the Lavender Symphony:
Share your experiences with Lavender with friends and family. Educate them about the benefits of this tranquil guardian. Encourage your social circle to explore the aromatic world of Lavender together, fostering a community dedicated to well-being.

3. Lavender Wellness Retreat:
Designate a day for a Lavender Wellness Retreat. Incorporate various Lavender rituals, from tea tastings to aromatherapy sessions, allowing a day of focused well-being. Share your retreat experience with others to inspire a collective journey toward aromatic tranquility.

4. Lavender in Daily Conversations:
Integrate Lavender into your daily conversations about well-being. Whether discussing stress relief or culinary adventures, introduce Lavender as a fragrant yet powerful ally. Promote awareness and understanding of its calming and antimicrobial charm.

5. Listen to Your Lavender Symphony:
Pay attention to the Lavender symphony within. Notice how incorporating Lavender into your routine influences your sleep and stress levels. Listen to the aromatic notes and the calming melody, and let your Lavender symphony guide you toward a healthier and more tranquil life.

Closing Tranquil Harmony:

As we conclude this chapter, envision Lavender not just as a pleasant scent but as the tranquil guardian that weaves through senses, carrying antimicrobial and calming notes. Let the lavender field, the nightly ritual, and the real-life examples inspire you to embrace the tranquil guardian of Lavender in your quest for vitality.

Sources:

1. Cavanagh, H. M. A., & Wilkinson, J. M. (2002). Biological activities of lavender essential oil. Phytotherapy Research, 16(4), 301–308.

2. Linck, V. M., da Silva, A. L., Figueiró, M., Caramão, E. B., Moreno, P. R. H., & Elisabetsky, E. (2010). Effects of inhaled linalool in anxiety, social interaction and aggressive behavior in mice. Phytomedicine, 17(8–9), 679–683.

3. Göbel, H., Schmidt, G., Dworschak, M., & Stolze, H. (1994). Essential plant oils and headache mechanisms. Phytomedicine, 1(2), 93–102.

29: Cranberry (Vaccinium macrocarpon): The Berry Defender - Anti-Urinary Tract Infection Marvel

Embark on a journey into the vibrant world of Cranberry, where the tiny berries of Vaccinium macrocarpon unveil their potent powers. In this chapter, we explore the enchanting realm of Cranberry, revealing its role as an extraordinary defender against urinary tract infections (UTIs), a berry marvel with the ability to safeguard your urinary well-being.

The Tart Prelude of Cranberry:
Picture a bog where Cranberry bushes thrive, and the tangy aroma of Cranberry Prelude fills the air. This isn't just a flavor; it's the essence of Cranberry, a natural melody carrying anti-UTI notes. Join us on this expedition into the heart of Cranberry, discovering its multifaceted role as a guardian against UTIs, fostering a symphony of urinary health.

Cranberry: Nature's Anti-UTI Marvel:
Cranberry isn't just a berry; it's nature's anti-UTI marvel, rich in compounds like proanthocyanidins. Laden with these elements, Cranberry becomes a guardian that not only tantalizes your taste buds but also stands as a formidable defender against urinary tract infections. Visualize it as the berry shield unlocking a world of urinary well-being.

Guardian Against UTIs:
Envision your urinary system as a delicate garden, and Cranberry as the vigilant guardian within. Scientific studies suggest that Cranberry, with its anti-adhesive properties, can act as a defender against UTIs.

Cranberry's symphony is not just a taste; it's a therapeutic anthem of urinary vitality ready to elevate your well-being.

Practical Tips for Cranberry Guardian:

1. Daily Cranberry Elixir:
Commence your Cranberry journey with a daily elixir. Incorporate pure Cranberry juice or a Cranberry supplement into your routine, unlocking not only its anti-UTI benefits but also supporting overall urinary health.

2. Cranberry-Infused Culinary Delights:
Immerse yourself in the culinary delights of Cranberry. Add fresh or dried Cranberries to your meals, enhancing not only the flavor but also infusing your dishes with anti-UTI richness.

3. Cranberry Wellness Hydration:
Embrace the wellness hydration of Cranberry. Create a refreshing Cranberry-infused water or herbal tea, allowing its anti-UTI properties to blend with your daily hydration routine and promote urinary health.

4. Cranberry Snack Ritual:
Infuse health into your snack ritual with Cranberries. Enjoy dried Cranberries as a snack, not only satisfying your taste buds but also reaping the anti-UTI benefits of this berry marvel.

5. Cranberry in Skincare Nectar:
Indulge in a Cranberry-infused skincare ritual. Create a Cranberry-infused facial mask or incorporate Cranberry

extracts into your skincare routine, unlocking not only its antioxidant properties but also promoting radiant skin from within.

Reflection Questions:

1. Reflect on your current understanding of urinary tract health. How open are you to exploring the role of Cranberry in enhancing this aspect of your well-being?
2. Consider Cranberry as nature's anti-UTI marvel. How might visualizing Cranberry's role as a berry shield influence your perception of its importance in your urinary health journey?
3. Envision your urinary system as a delicate garden. In what ways can Cranberry actively contribute to guarding against UTIs, fostering a protective and vibrant relationship between your lifestyle and urinary well-being?
4. Reflect on the practical tips for Cranberry guardian. How might incorporating these rituals and recipes into your daily life positively impact your well-being?
5. Think about the guardian role of Cranberry against UTIs. How does the knowledge of its protective properties empower you to embrace a Cranberry-inspired approach to urinary vitality?

Real-Life Examples:

Example 1: Maya's Daily Cranberry Elixir:
Meet Maya, who starts each day with a glass of pure Cranberry juice. This daily elixir not only delights her taste buds but also supports her urinary health, showcasing the simplicity of integrating wellness into daily practices.

Example 2: Raj's Cranberry-Infused Culinary Delights:
Raj, a culinary enthusiast, adds fresh Cranberries to his meals. Whether in salads or sauces, Cranberries enhance not only the flavor but also infuse his dishes with anti-UTI richness. Raj's culinary delights with Cranberry highlight the versatility of this berry in enhancing daily meals.

Example 3: Olivia's Cranberry Wellness Hydration:
Olivia embraces the wellness hydration of Cranberry. Creating a refreshing Cranberry-infused water, she not only quenches her thirst but also supports her urinary health with every sip. Olivia's hydration ritual with Cranberry exemplifies the fusion of nature and daily wellness.

Example 4: Ethan's Cranberry Snack Ritual:
Ethan infuses health into his snack ritual with Cranberries. Enjoying dried Cranberries as a snack, he not only satisfies his taste buds but also reaps the anti-UTI benefits of this berry marvel. Ethan's snack ritual with Cranberry showcases the adaptability of this berry in promoting health.

Example 5: Zoe's Cranberry in Skincare Nectar:
Zoe indulges in a Cranberry-infused skincare ritual. Incorporating Cranberry extracts into her skincare routine not only adds antioxidant properties but also promotes radiant skin from within. Zoe's skincare nectar with Cranberry highlights the integration of therapeutic practices into daily self-care.

The Berry Defender: Cranberry:

Cranberry isn't just a berry; it's the defender that weaves through senses, carrying anti-UTI notes. The Cranberry bog, the daily elixir, and the real-life examples of individuals embracing Cranberry in various forms showcase its potential to positively transform your urinary well-being.

Actionable Advice:

1. Cranberry Wellness Journal:
Create a Cranberry Wellness Journal to document your journey. Record your experiences, feelings, and any noticeable changes in your urinary health as you incorporate Cranberry into your routine. This journal becomes a personal guide on your berry-infused path to vitality.

2. Share the Cranberry Symphony:
Share your experiences with Cranberry with friends and family. Educate them about the benefits of this berry defender. Encourage your social circle to explore the world of Cranberry together, fostering a community dedicated to urinary well-being.

3. Cranberry Wellness Retreat:
Designate a day for a Cranberry Wellness Retreat. Incorporate various Cranberry rituals, from culinary adventures to skincare sessions, allowing a day of focused well-being. Share your retreat experience with others to inspire a collective journey toward berry-infused vitality.

4. Cranberry in Daily Conversations:
Integrate Cranberry into your daily conversations about well-being. Whether discussing hydration or culinary adventures, introduce Cranberry as a tangy yet powerful ally. Promote awareness and understanding of its anti-UTI charm.

5. Listen to Your Cranberry Symphony:
Pay attention to the Cranberry symphony within. Notice how incorporating Cranberry into your routine influences your urinary well-being. Listen to the tangy notes and the protective melody, and let your Cranberry symphony guide you toward a healthier and more vibrant life.

Closing Berry Harmony:

As we conclude this chapter, envision Cranberry not just as a tart flavor but as the berry defender that weaves through senses, carrying anti-UTI notes. Let the Cranberry bog, the daily elixir, and the real-life examples inspire you to embrace the berry defender of Cranberry in your quest for urinary vitality.

Sources:
1. Howell, A. B., & Foxman, B. (2002). Cranberry juice and adhesion of antibiotic-resistant uropathogens. Journal of the American Medical Association, 287(23), 3082–3083.
2. Jepson, R. G., & Williams, G. (2012). Cranberries for preventing urinary tract infections. Cochrane Database of Systematic Reviews, 10, CD001321.
3. Howell, A. B. (2002). Cranberry proanthocyanidins and the maintenance of urinary tract health. Critical

Reviews in Food Science and Nutrition, 42(suppl 3), 273–278.

30: Colloidal Silver: The Elemental Finale - An Antimicrobial Conclusion

As we embark on the final chapter of our journey through the verdant landscapes of natural antibiotics, we find ourselves at the threshold of an elemental revelation—Colloidal Silver, the concluding note in our symphony of natural remedies. In this chapter, we delve into the unique properties of Colloidal Silver, a silver lining that crowns our exploration with its antimicrobial brilliance, bringing our odyssey to a resonant and powerful conclusion.

The Elemental Overture of Colloidal Silver:
Imagine a minute suspension of silver particles, shimmering in a liquid medium, creating an elemental overture that resonates with healing potential. This isn't just a solution; it's the essence of Colloidal Silver, a natural harmony carrying antimicrobial notes. Join us on this final expedition into the heart of Colloidal Silver, discovering its multifaceted role as an elemental defender against a spectrum of microbes.

Colloidal Silver: Nature's Antimicrobial Emissary:
Colloidal Silver isn't just a liquid; it's nature's antimicrobial emissary, composed of tiny silver particles suspended in a solution. Laden with these elements, Colloidal Silver becomes a guardian that not only shimmers in its simplicity but also stands as a formidable defender against a broad spectrum of microbes. Visualize it as the elemental shield unlocking a world of microbial balance.

Guardian Against Microbial Imbalance:
Envision your body as a delicate ecosystem, and Colloidal Silver as the vigilant guardian within. Scientific studies suggest that Colloidal Silver, with its unique antimicrobial properties, can act as a defender against various microbes. Colloidal Silver's symphony is not just a metallic taste; it's a therapeutic anthem of balance ready to elevate your well-being.

Practical Tips for Colloidal Silver Guardian:

1. Elemental Daily Supplement:
Commence your Colloidal Silver journey with a daily supplement. Incorporate a high-quality Colloidal Silver supplement into your routine, unlocking not only its antimicrobial benefits but also supporting overall microbial balance.

2. Colloidal Silver Infused Hydration:
Embrace the hydration of Colloidal Silver. Create a refreshing Colloidal Silver-infused water, allowing its antimicrobial properties to blend with your daily hydration routine and promote overall microbial health.

3. Colloidal Silver Topical Elixir:
Indulge in a Colloidal Silver-infused topical elixir. Create a simple spray or gel with Colloidal Silver, incorporating its antimicrobial properties into your skincare routine, promoting balance and wellness.

4. Colloidal Silver in Environmental Harmony:
Infuse Colloidal Silver into your environmental harmony. Use Colloidal Silver as a natural disinfectant for surfaces, promoting a clean and

balanced living space that supports microbial equilibrium.

5. Colloidal Silver Wellness Ritual:
Make Colloidal Silver a part of your wellness ritual. Whether as a supplement, topical elixir, or environmental disinfectant, integrate Colloidal Silver into your daily practices, fostering microbial balance and overall well-being.

Reflection Questions:

1. Reflect on your journey through the realms of natural antibiotics. How has the exploration of various remedies enriched your understanding of health and well-being?
2. Consider Colloidal Silver as the elemental finale. How might visualizing Colloidal Silver as an antimicrobial emissary influence your perception of its importance in maintaining microbial balance?
3. Envision your body as a delicate ecosystem. In what ways can Colloidal Silver actively contribute to guarding against microbial imbalance, fostering a protective and vibrant relationship between your lifestyle and overall microbial health?
4. Reflect on the practical tips for Colloidal Silver guardian. How might incorporating these rituals and recipes into your daily life positively impact your well-being?
5. Think about the guardian role of Colloidal Silver against microbial imbalance. How does the knowledge of its protective properties empower you to embrace a Colloidal Silver-inspired approach to microbial vitality?

Real-Life Examples:

Example 1: Alex's Elemental Daily Supplement:
Meet Alex, who starts each day with a high-quality Colloidal Silver supplement. This daily elemental supplement not only brings simplicity to his routine but also supports his overall microbial balance, showcasing the ease of integrating wellness into daily practices.

Example 2: Morgan's Colloidal Silver Infused Hydration:
Morgan embraces the hydration of Colloidal Silver. Creating a refreshing Colloidal Silver-infused water, she not only quenches her thirst but also supports her overall microbial health with every sip. Morgan's hydration ritual with Colloidal Silver exemplifies the fusion of nature and daily wellness.

Example 3: Taylor's Colloidal Silver Topical Elixir:
Taylor indulges in a Colloidal Silver-infused topical elixir. Creating a simple spray or gel with Colloidal Silver, she incorporates its antimicrobial properties into her skincare routine, promoting balance and wellness. Taylor's skincare elixir with Colloidal Silver showcases the adaptability of this elemental solution in enhancing daily self-care.

Example 4: Jordan's Colloidal Silver in Environmental Harmony:
Jordan infuses Colloidal Silver into his environmental harmony. Using Colloidal Silver as a natural disinfectant for surfaces, he promotes a clean and balanced living space that supports microbial equilibrium. Jordan's environmental harmony with Colloidal Silver highlights its role

beyond personal well-being, extending to the spaces we inhabit.

Example 5: Riley's Colloidal Silver Wellness Ritual:
Riley makes Colloidal Silver a part of her wellness ritual. Whether as a supplement, topical elixir, or environmental disinfectant, she integrates Colloidal Silver into her daily practices, fostering microbial balance and overall well-being. Riley's wellness ritual with Colloidal Silver exemplifies a holistic approach to health.

The Elemental Finale: Colloidal Silver:

Colloidal Silver isn't just a solution; it's the elemental finale that weaves through senses, carrying antimicrobial notes. The shimmering suspension, the daily supplement, and the real-life examples of individuals embracing Colloidal Silver in various forms showcase its potential to positively transform your microbial vitality.

Actionable Advice:

1. Colloidal Silver Wellness Journal:
Create a Colloidal Silver Wellness Journal to document your journey. Record your experiences, feelings, and any noticeable changes in your overall microbial health as you incorporate Colloidal Silver into your routine. This journal becomes a personal guide on your elemental path to vitality.

2. Share the Colloidal Silver Symphony:
Share your experiences with Colloidal Silver with friends and family. Educate them about the benefits of this elemental solution. Encourage your social

circle to explore the world of Colloidal Silver together, fostering a community dedicated to microbial well-being.

3. Colloidal Silver Wellness Retreat:
Designate a day for a Colloidal Silver Wellness Retreat. Incorporate various Colloidal Silver rituals, from supplement intake to skincare sessions, allowing a day of focused well-being. Share your retreat experience with others to inspire a collective journey toward elemental vitality.

4. Colloidal Silver in Daily Conversations:
Integrate Colloidal Silver into your daily conversations about well-being. Whether discussing hydration or environmental harmony, introduce Colloidal Silver as a shimmering yet powerful ally. Promote awareness and understanding of its antimicrobial charm.

5. Listen to Your Colloidal Silver Symphony:
Pay attention to the Colloidal Silver symphony within. Notice how incorporating Colloidal Silver into your routine influences your microbial well-being. Listen to the elemental notes and the balancing melody, and let your Colloidal Silver symphony guide you toward a healthier and more vibrant life.

Closing Elemental Harmony:

As we conclude this final chapter and the entire journey through the realms of natural antibiotics, envision Colloidal Silver not just as a shimmering solution but as the elemental finale that weaves through senses, carrying antimicrobial notes. Let the elemental suspension, the daily supplement, and the real-life examples inspire you to embrace the elemental finale of Colloidal Silver in your quest for vibrant microbial vitality.

Sources:
1. Morones-Ramirez, J. R., Winkler, J. A., Spina, C. S., & Collins, J. J. (2013). Silver enhances antibiotic activity against gram-negative bacteria. Science Translational Medicine, 5(190), 190ra81.
2. Lansdown, A. B. (2006). Silver in health care: antimicrobial effects and safety in use. Current Problems in Dermatology, 33, 17–34.